Study Guide and
Computerized Learning Resource
to Accompany

NURSING RESEARCH

Methods, Critical Appraisal, and Utilization

Study Guide and Computerized Learning Resource to Accompany

NURSING RESEARCH
Methods, Critical Appraisal, and Utilization

Kathleen Rose-Grippa, PhD, RN
Professor and Director
School of Nursing
Ohio University
Athens, Ohio

Mary Jo Gorney-Lucero, PhD, RN
Professor and Undergraduate Coordinator
College of Nursing
San Jose State University
San Jose, California

Computerized Learning Resource by
Barbara S. Thomas, PhD
Professor
College of Nursing
University of Iowa
Iowa City, Iowa

THIRD EDITION

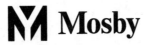 Mosby

St. Louis Baltimore Boston Chicago London Madrid Philadelphia Sydney Toronto

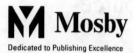
Dedicated to Publishing Excellence

Executive Editor: N. Darlene Como
Senior Developmental Editor: Laurie Sparks
Manuscript Editor: Susan Warrington
Design and Layout: Ken Wendling

THIRD EDITION

Printed in the United States of America

Mosby-Year Book, Inc.
11830 Westline Industrial Drive
St. Louis, Missouri 63146

International Standard Book Number 0-8151-5628-6

Contributors

Sharon Denham, MSN, RN
Assistant Professor
School of Nursing
Ohio University
Athens, Ohio

Elizabeth O. Dietz, EdD, RN, CS
Professor, Nurse Practitioner
School of Nursing
San Jose State University
San Jose, California

Ann Marttinen Doordan, PhD, CRRN
Associate Professor, Advanced Placement Coordinator
Director, Institute for Nursing Research and Practice
School of Nursing
San Jose State University
San Jose, California

Mary Jo Gorney-Lucero, PhD, RN
Professor and Undergraduate Coordinator
College of Nursing
San Jose State University
San Jose, California

Sharon S. Mullen, PhD, RN
Assistant Professor
School of Nursing
Ohio University
Athens, Ohio

Kay L. Palmer, MSN, RN, CRRN
Associate Professor
School of Nursing
Old Dominion University
Norfolk, Virginia

Mary M. Reeve, EdD, RN
Associate Professor, Curriculum Coordinator
School of Nursing
San Jose State University
San Jose, California

Kathleen Rose-Grippa, PhD, RN
Professor and Director
School of Nursing
Ohio University
Athens, Ohio

Table of Contents

INTRODUCTION

As we stated in the first edition: What an exciting time to be a nurse! The clinically relevant research studies continue to increase and even more nurses are participating in research. As the number and variety of studies expand, it becomes increasingly important for nurses to evaluate the value and clinical significance of those studies published. The activities in this study guide are designed to assist you in gaining these skills. May your clients and fellow professionals benefit from your persistence, your hard work, and your thinking.

GENERAL DIRECTIONS

1. Do each chapter and the activities in it sequentially. The study guide is designed so that the knowledge gained in Activity 1 will be helpful in completing Activities 2, 3, and so on.

   The activities are designed to give you the opportunity to apply the knowledge learned and actually use it to solve problems, thus gaining the increased confidence that comes only from working through each chapter.

2. Follow the specific directions that precede each activity. Be certain that you have the resources needed to complete the activity you start.

3. Do the posttest after all activities have been completed. Check with your instructor for the answers. If you answer 85% of the questions correctly, you can feel confident that you have grasped the essential material presented in the chapter.

4. Clarify any questions, confusion, or concerns with your instructors, or write the editors of the study guide.

SELECTED ANSWERS

Answers in a workbook such as this are not "cut and dried," as they might be in a math workbook. Many times, you are asked to make a judgement call about a particular problem. If your judgement differs from the authors' judgement, review the criteria that you used to make your decision. Decide if you followed a logical progression of steps to reach your decision. If not, rework the activity. If the process you followed appears logical, and you still arrive at a different answer, be aware that even experts are not always in agreement on many of the judgement calls in nursing research. There are many "gray" areas. If, on the average, you are in 85% agreement with the authors, you are on the right track and should feel confident with your level of expertise.

Don't forget the areas of disagreement, though. These are excellent starting points for your dialogue with other nurses about specific research studies. It is the responsibility of members of a profession to critique and dialogue about important professional issues. When basing your practice on new or different techniques or methods based on research, you need to analyze this innovation critically with your colleagues. Does the innovation "fit" your practice setting? Only after these dialogues will you and your colleagues be ready to contemplate seriously the adoption of research-based findings in your practice settings. Happy discourse!

CHAPTER

1

The Role of Research in Nursing

INTRODUCTION

One goal of this chapter in the study guide is to assist you in reviewing the material presented in Chapter 1 of the text written by LoBiondo-Wood and Haber. A second and more fundamental goal is to provide you with an opportunity to begin to practice the role of a critical consumer of research. Succeeding chapters in this workbook fine-tune your ability to evaluate research studies critically.

LEARNING OBJECTIVES

On completion of this chapter, the student should be able to do the following:

- Identify the research roles associated with each of the educational levels of nurses.
- Recognize titles and names associated with significant events in the history of nursing research.
- Identify nursing's role in future trends in research.

ACTIVITY 1

Match the term in Column B with the appropriate phrase in Column A.

Column A

1. __C__ systematic inquiry into possible relationships among particular phenomena
2. __B__ one who reads critically and applies research findings in nursing practice
3. __D__ examines the effects of nursing care on patient outcomes in a systematic process
4. __A__ critically evaluates a research report's content based on a set of criteria to evaluate the scientific merit for application
5. __E__ theoretical or pure research that generates tests and expands theories that explain phenomena

Column B

a. critique
b. consumer
c. research
d. clinical research
e. basic research

Check your answers with those in Appendix A, Chapter 1.

ACTIVITY 2

Listed below are specific research activities. Using the American Nurses' Association (ANA) guidelines, indicate which group of nurses has the primary responsibility for each activity. Use the abbreviations from the key provided.

KEY: A = associate degree   C = master's degree
       B = baccalaureate degree   D = doctoral degree

1. __D__   Design research studies
2. __B__   Identify nursing problems needing investigation
3. __C__   Assist others in applying nursing's scientific knowledge
4. __D__   Develop methods of scientific inquiry
5. __A__   Assist in data collection activities
6. __B__   Be a knowledgeable consumer of research
7. __A__   Demonstrate an awareness of value of nursing research
8. __C__   Collaborate with an experienced researcher in proposal development, data analysis and interpretation

Check your answers with those in Appendix A, Chapter 1.

ACTIVITY 3

Work the following crossword puzzle as you would any other crossword puzzle. Note that if more than one word is needed in an answer, there will be no blank spaces between the words of the name or phrase. Refer to the text for help.

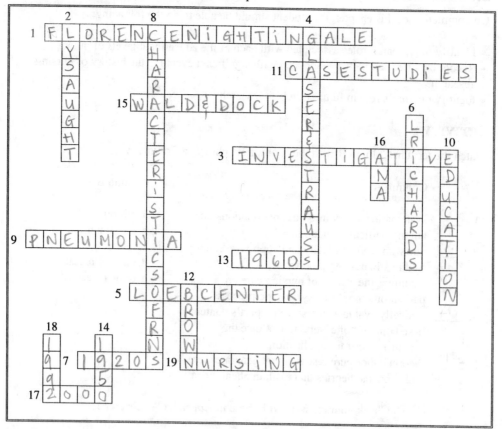

Across

1. Collected and analyzed data on the health status of the British Army during the Crimean War.
3. In 1981 the ANA published guidelines for the role of the nurse in research. What synonym for the word *research* was used in the title?
5. Lydia Hall's research led to the creation of this totally nurse-run health care facility.
7. Earliest nursing research course taught in this decade (numeral).
9. One of the first topics of clinically oriented research.
11. The 1920s saw much of this type of research published in the *American Journal of Nursing (AJN)*.
13. A decade of increased emphasis on practice-oriented research (numeral).
15. The research of _____ and _____ led to New York City's hiring of school nurses.
17. *Healthy People* _____ published by the Public Health Service (numeral).
19. National Center for _____ Research established in 1986 at NIH.

Down

2. _____Report, published in 1970, concluded that more practice-oriented and education-oriented research was necessary.
4. They studied aspects of thanatology, the care of dying patients, and their caretakers. (Use ampersand [&] between names.)
6. First nurse to keep systematic written records of client care (such records are critical to retrospective research).
8. Focus of nursing research in the 1950s.
10. Focus of nursing research between 1900 and 1950.
12. _____Report emphasized the need for nursing education to move into the university.
14. First year of the decade in which the *Journal of Nursing Research* was first published (numeral).
16. This organization sponsored the First Nursing Research Conference in 1967.
18. Year *Clinical Practice Guidelines: Urinary Incontinence, Acute Pain Management and Pressure Ulcers* published by AHCPR (numeral).

Check your answers with those in Appendix A, Chapter 1.

ACTIVITY 4

1. Examine the three articles that are in the appendices of the text. What is the educational preparation of the persons responsible for each study? List the degrees (RN, BSN, M.S., Ph.D., or D.N.Sc.) of each author next to the author's name. Remember, this information is usually found in the short biographical paragraph on the first page or at the end of the article.

   a. Stewart Fahs __RN, MSN__   Kinney __RN, DNSc__

   b. Grey __PhD__   Cameron __MS, RN__   Thurber __PhD, RN__

   c. Hutchison __RN, DNSc__   Bahr __RN, PhD__

2. In what way does this information regarding the educational preparation of the researcher influence your thinking about the study? Before drawing any conclusions, answer the following questions:

   a. Is the first author's education preparation at the doctoral level?   No

Appendix A: Yes No

Appendix B: Yes No

Appendix C: Yes No

(The general assumption is that the first author carries the major responsibility for the research.)

b. If there are other authors and they do not have master's or doctoral degrees, what evidence is there that they are working on such a degree?

Appendix A _____

Appendix B _____

Appendix C _____

c. Are any of the authors associated with a college or university? Are their academic titles listed? Briefly describe below.

Appendix A _____

Appendix B _____

Appendix C _____

(Remember, one usually begins as a lecturer or an assistant professor, then becomes an associate professor, with the highest academic rank being professor.)

d. Were any of the studies funded by external funding agencies? Write below which study and which agency. This would indicate that the research proposal had been reviewed by an external source and deemed of enough merit to received funding to complete.

_____

_____

_____

_____

Check your answers with those in Appendix A, Chapter 1.

ACTIVITY 5

The Department of Health and Human Services published *Healthy People 2000* in 1992. The report is a compilation of 22 expert working groups who specified as one of their objectives "to reduce physical abuse directed at women by male partners to no more than 27 per 1,000

couples." One example of the way nursing is helping to achieve this objective is through studies and publications such as the 1993 *Nursing Research* article "Physical and emotional
abuse in pregnancy: a comparison of adult and teen-age women" by Parker. Other ways nursing and nurse researchers are helping to address this objective are:

a. _continuing to conduct research on the topic of abuse in_

b. _developing theoretical perspectives_

c. _conducting synthesis conferences into the area of abuse in_

d. _using nsg research studies to assist in legislative_

Check your answers with those in Appendix A, Chapter 1.

POSTTEST

1. Listed below are descriptions of research activities being carried out by nurses. Indicate in
   the space in front of each description whether the action is most appropriate to:
   A = an associate degree prepared nurse
   B = a baccalaureate degree prepared nurse
   C = a master's prepared nurse
   D = a doctorally prepared nurse

   a. __B__ Provide expert consulting to a unit that is considering changing the unit's
   practice on the care of decubitus ulcers based on the results from a series of
   studies

   b. __A__ Take and record the blood pressures of hypertensive clients during their month-
   ly visits to the clinic as part of a study on the effects of contingency contracting
   by a nurse researcher

   c. __C__ To understand and critically appraise research studies to discriminate whether
   a study is provocative or whether the findings have sufficient support to be
   considered for utilization

   d. __D__ Design and conduct research studies to expand nursing knowledge, such as the
   Anderson study, "The parenting profile assessment: Screening for child abuse"

2. Match the term in Column B with the appropriate phrase in Column A. Not all terms from
   Column B will be used.

Column A	Column B
1. __D__ first nursing doctoral program began at Teacher's College, Columbia University 1924	a. 1910-1919
2. __E__ National Center for Nursing Research established at NIH	b. mid and late 19th century
3. __B__ Nightingale studied mortality rates of British in Crimean War 1855	c. 1992
4. __A__ American Nurses' Association established 1912	d. 1920-1929
5. __F__ *Nursing Research* publication began 1952	e. 1986
	f. 1952
	g. 1900
	h. 2000

The answers to the posttest are in the Instructor's Resource Manual. Please check with your
instructor for these answers.

REFERENCES

Anderson, C. (1993). The parenting profile assessment: Screening for child abuse. *Applied Nursing Research*, 6(1), 31-38.

Parker, B., et al. (1993). Physical and emotional abuse in pregnancy: A comparison of adult and teen-age women. *Nursing Research*, 42(3).

CHAPTER

2

The Scientific Approach to the Research Process

INTRODUCTION

In this chapter you are given a series of exercises that introduce you to both the research process and the scientific process and allow you to compare each with the nursing process. Once you have a clear understanding of both processes, you can critique studies to determine if they adhere to the philosophy of these processes. If you determine that a study does adhere to the correct protocol, then you may decide that the information learned from the study is of sufficient merit to consider incorporating the results into your practice.

LEARNING OBJECTIVES

On completion of this chapter, the student should be able to do the following:

• Match key term with the appropriate definition.
• Compare two methods of knowledge development: structured and unstructured.
• Apply the inductive and deductive reasoning processes to specific clinical examples.
• Compare and contrast the research process and the nursing process.

ACTIVITY 1

Chapter 2 of the text discusses a variety of methods for generating human/nursing knowledge. It separates knowledge development into two categories: unstructured and structured. For each of the terms below put a **U** for Unstructured or an **S** for a Structured method of generating knowledge.

1. _____ Research
2. _____ Tradition
3. _____ Authority
4. _____ Nursing Process
5. _____ Deduction
6. _____ Intuition

Check your answers with those in Appendix A, Chapter 2.

ACTIVITY 2

Match the term in Column B with the appropriate phrase in Column A.

Column A	Column B
1. _____ using research to predict future outcomes and relationships	a. theory
2. _____ a systematic and controlled complex process	b. hypothesis
3. _____ moves from general to the particular	c. inductive reasoning
4. _____ basic principles assumed to be true	d. assumption
5. _____ provides a framework from which hypotheses are tested	e. deductive reasoning
6. _____ moves from the particular to the general	f. research consumer
7. _____ has the responsibility to evaluate research approaches	g. generalization
8. _____ statement of relationship between two or more variables	h. scientific approach
9. _____ a process of seeking knowledge based on either an intuitive or a scientific approach	i. intuition
10. _____ a problem-solving method based on innate knowledge	j. research

Check your answers with those in Appendix A, Chapter 2.

ACTIVITY 3

Read the following situation. Mentally attempt to define and study the problem first from an inductive and then from deductive perspective. Then label each of the processes that follows as to whether the problem solving steps show an attempt at study from an inductive or deductive approach.

Case Situation

You are working on a surgical unit. There are many female patients on this unit who return from hysterectomies with a foley catheter in place. From your casual observations, it appears that the most frequent postoperative problem these patients have is the inability to void when the catheter is removed. The result is a cycle of catheter removal, difficulty in voiding, and re-catheterization, which in turn leads to increased susceptibility to bladder infections and prolonged hospitalization.

Process 1

a. You begin to observe all hysterectomy patients in a systematic manner.
b. You develop a checklist for your observations to make sure that they are similar.
c. You attempt to look at a number of variables to determine if there were any differences.
d. After a period of data collection or a number of patients on whom you collected data, you might try to organize your information in a meaningful way (e.g., develop graphs or charts).
e. You use the information you have gathered to write a proposal or to approach a nurse researcher about the need for a study in the area.

f. You write an article that describes your observations as an incident specific to one setting and one group of patients.

Circle either **inductive** or **deductive**, correctly labeling the process just described.

Process 2
a. You would search for a theory that explains this phenomenon.
b. You or an appropriately prepared nurse researcher colleague develop hypotheses based on this theory.
c. You develop a research proposal to test these hypotheses.
d. You or your colleague conduct the research study.
e. You discuss and draw conclusions about the data collected in the research study.
f. The conclusions drawn might give you information about the phenomenon in question that you may be able to use to design a clinical intervention.

Circle either **inductive** or **deductive**, correctly labeling the process just described.

Check your answers with those in Appendix A, Chapter 2.

ACTIVITY 4

Following is a list of the steps in the research process and the nursing process.

Research Process
1. Formulate and delimit the problem
2. Review related literature
3. Develop a theoretical framework
4. Identify the variables
5. Formulate hypotheses
6. Select a research design
7. Collect the data
8. Analyze the data
9. Interpret the results
10. Communicate findings

Nursing Process
1. Assessment
2. Planning
3. Implementation
4. Evaluation

a. Draw lines between the steps that are the same.

b. Circle the steps in either process that do not have a similar step in the other process.

c. How are the two processes similar?

_____

_____

d. How are two processes different?

_____

_____

Check your answers with those in Appendix A, Chapter 2.

1. List five sources of Nursing Knowledge.

   a. _____

   b. _____

   c. _____

   d. _____

   e. _____

2. There are two major ways to approach either a clinical or a research problem. One way is the inductive approach based on discovery through observations of a particular set of events and summarization of this information. A second way to approach a problem is deductively, i.e., using the theory-test approach to look from the general to the specific.

   List the advantages and disadvantages of each of these styles of logical thinking.

   Advantages

   Inductive: Deductive:

   _____   _____

   _____   _____

   _____   _____

   Disadvantages

   Inductive: Deductive:

   _____   _____

   _____   _____

   _____   _____

3. Put a **T** (for True) or an **F** (for False) in front of the following statements:

   a. _____ As research consumers, nurses are asked to judge why and how ideas were generated and related.

   b. _____ The scientific approach is based on unstructured intuition and trial and error methods.

c. _____ The philosophical viewpoints of the researcher influence the direction of the research.

d. _____ It is appropriate for a nurse to question a traditional approach to a nursing practice by reviewing related literature and consulting experts.

e. _____ The research process begins with developing a theoretical framework.

The answers to the posttest are in the Instructor's Resource Manual. Please check with your instructor for these answers.

REFERENCE

LoBiondo-Wood, G. and Haber, J. (1994). *Nursing research: Methods, critical appraisal and utilization* (3rd ed.) St. Louis: Mosby-Year Book, Inc.

3

The Evolution of Research: From Science to Practice

INTRODUCTION

Nurses, like other health care practitioners, are obligated to improve the care they deliver. As researchers work to expand nursing's knowledge of those factors that influence nursing care, clinicians need to be reading research and thinking, "How can I use this information to improve the care I (or this unit or this agency) deliver?" The following activities will help you consider answers to that question.

LEARNING OBJECTIVES

On completion of this chapter, the student should be able to do the following:

- Discuss the contribution of selected research findings to clinical practice and patient outcomes.
- Identify the application of selected findings to actual clinical practice.
- In a selected research study determine the applicability of findings to a selected clinical practice situation.
- Identify factors in a clinical environment that facilitate the use of research findings.
- Identify factors in a clinical environment that act as barriers to the use of research findings.
- Utilize strategies to promote clinical research studies in selected case situations.

ACTIVITY 1

Match the term in Column B with the appropriate phrase in Column A. Not all terms from Column B will be used.

Column A

1. __F__ a receiver for programs beamed from other agencies which allows you to participate in a program occurring at some other site

2. __B__ a systematic method of implementing a sound research-based innovation in clinical practice, evaluating the outcome and sharing the knowledge through the process of research dissemination

Column B

a. uplink
b. research utilization
c. replication
d. barrier to research utilization
e. NUCARE (Nursing Care Research)
f. downlink

3. _A_ the ability of your agency to broadcast conferences in which you may be able to participate

4. _E_ online research conference that allows nurses to share nursing care information and use technology to facilitate more nursing research

5. _D_ research articles in journals that use "jargon specific to a small number of insiders"

Check your answers with those in Appendix A, Chapter 3.

ACTIVITY 2

Fill in the blanks in the following sentences.

1. Many of the tasks of nursing care are done in a certain manner because of the "sacred cows" of ___tradition___, ___authority___, and ___trial & error___

2. One of the first research utilization efforts was done by _____.

3. To help clinicians utilize research, the WICHEN project recommended that researchers include _____ in the reports.

4. All nurses should _____ research.

5. Research dissemination and utilization is a major responsibility of _____ nurse.

6. The two greatest barriers to research utilization are _____ and _____.

7. Three methods I can do personally to increase research utilization are _____, _____, and _____.

8. It is essential that nursing as a profession provide evidence that it does make a difference because:

   a. _____

   b. _____

   c. _____

9. Changes in nursing practice _____ (should/should not) occur as a result of one study.

10. Nursing research should be conducted to _____.

11. Name two major private foundations that fund nursing research.

    a. _____

    b. _____

12. List two priorities for research by the NCNR (National Center for Nursing Research).

    a. _____

    b. _____

Check your answers with those in Appendix A, Chapter 3.

ACTIVITY 3

1. Review the Stewart Fahs and Kinney study (1991) in Appendix A of the text to discuss what the findings from the study could mean in your clinical practice.

2. Utilize the CURN criteria found on page 8 to review the study by Stewart Fahs and Kinney in Appendix A of the text. Identify for each of the following criterion one or more points that support your decision that the study by Stewart Fahs and Kinney meets or does not meet the criterion:

    a. Scientific merit

    _____

    _____

    _____

    _____

    b. Replicability

    _____

    _____

    _____

    _____

c. Relevance to practice

_____

_____

_____

_____

d. Importance as a client problem

_____

_____

_____

_____

e. Feasibility for nurses to implement

_____

_____

_____

_____

f. Risk-benefit ratio

_____

_____

_____

_____

3. Utilize the Stetler/Marram model for Application of Research Findings (found in Figure 3-1 and Table 3-1 of the textbook) to review the Stewart Fahs and Kinney research study.

The following key words will help you think this through.

Phase I: Validation

a. Scientific merit _____

_____

_____

b. Significance for practice _____

_____

_____

c. Strength of study _____

d. Should we proceed to Phase II? _____

Phase II: Comparative Evaluation

a. Substantiating evidence _____

_____

_____

b. Fitness of setting _____

_____

_____

c. Basis for practice _____

_____

_____

d. Feasibility _____

_____

_____

Phase III: Decision Making

a. Nonapplication? _____

_____

b. Cognitive application? _____

_____

c. Action application? _____

_____

4. Find the boxes on page 72 in the text. Both contain thought questions.
Answer the questions in the upper box if you are a student who is not licensed as an RN.
Answer the questions in the lower box if you are a licensed RN taking this course.

Check your answers with those in Appendix A, Chapter 3.

POSTTEST

1. All nurses must _____ research.

2. True False   The research process ends when the study is completed.

3. True False   Nursing can provide evidence that it makes a difference in providing quality care through research.

4. Some of the results from research include all of the following except:
   a. Enhances professional image.
   b. Helps find cost-effective outcomes.
   c. Can provide answers to all practice questions.

5. True False   One of the major goals of the WICHEN research utilization project was to facilitate the interaction between researchers and practitioners.

6. True False   The greatest barriers to utilization of nursing research as perceived by nurses lie within the setting in which they work.

7. List three barriers, personal or professional, to the utilization of research findings.

   a. _____

   b. _____

   c. _____

8. List three educational or communication barriers to the utilization of nursing research.

   a. _____

   b. _____

   c. _____

9. True   False   Research competence is required only at the master's level of nursing preparation and above.

10. True   False   An external driving force for utilization of research is the American Nurses' Association.

11. Nurse researchers must utilize language that is _____ by nurses who work directly with patients.

12. Private organizations are funding all of the following research initiatives except:
    a. Research dealing with early discharge and home care programs.
    b. Strategies to increase compliance with medication usage in hypertensive young adults.
    c. Collaborative studies emphasizing methods to decrease the risk factors with heart disease.
    d. Effective methods of teaching nursing theory.

13. True   False   Nursing Leaders are pushing to have The Center for Nursing Research be converted to a National Institute of Nursing Research equal in status to the other National Health Institutes.

14. True   False   The unit-based research committee could include staff nurses functioning as investigators.

15. True   False   Students should share information from their research projects with the staff who were involved.

16. True   False   Researchers need to be close to clinical practice issues.

The answers to the posttest are in the Instructor's Resource Manual. Please check with your instructor for these answers.

REFERENCE

Stewart Fahs, P. S. and Kinney, M. R. (1991). The abdomen, thigh, and arm as sites for subcutaneous sodium heparin injections. *Nursing Research*, 40(4), 204-207.

CHAPTER

4

Overview of the Research Process: A Critical Reading Perspective

INTRODUCTION

Tools are needed for whatever task one sets out to do. Sometimes the tools are relatively simple and concrete, e.g., a pencil. Other times the tools are abstract and more difficult to describe. The tools you need to critically consider research fit into the abstract tool category. They are tools of the mind, i.e., critical thinking and critical reading tools. The following activities are designed to help you recognize and use these tools.

LEARNING OBJECTIVES

On completion of this chapter, the student should be able to do the following:

- Identify the characteristics of critical thinking.
- Identify the components of critical reading.
- Use the components of critical thinking and critical reading on selected passages.

ACTIVITY 1

Complete each item with the appropriate word or phrase from the text.

1. Critical thinking is a/an _____ (rational or irrational) process.

2. Critical reading requires the reader to participate in a _____ with the writer.

3. Another way of stating this reader-writer relationship is: The reader looks at the world

   from the _____.

4. Name the four stages of understanding that can be achieved through critical reading.

   a. _____

   b. _____

   c. _____

d. _____

5. What is the minimum number of readings of a research article recommended in the text?

_____

Check your answers with those in Appendix A, Chapter 4.

ACTIVITY 2

Match the term in Column B with the appropriate phrase in Column A. Terms from Column B will be used more than once.

Column A   Column B

1. _____ to get a general sense of the material   a. critical thinking
2. _____ requires use of research text and dictionary   b. critical reading
3. _____ constructive skepticism
4. _____ to understand each aspect of a study
5. _____ rational process
6. _____ thinking about your own thinking

Check your answers with those in Appendix A, Chapter 4.

ACTIVITY 3

The process of critical reading has four components. Each component has several steps. In each of the following four exercises, the steps in a given component are presented in a scrambled order. You are to rearrange each set into the appropriate order.

1. Preliminary understanding

Scrambled order:

Review old and new terms
Write key variables at the top of the page
Read the abstract closely
Highlight or underline main steps of research process
Skim the complete article

Appropriate order:

a. _____

b. _____

c. _____

d. _____

e. _____

2. Comprehensive understanding

Scrambled order:

State main idea in own words
Read additional sources as necessary
Review unfamiliar terms
Write cues, concept relations, etc., on copy of article

Appropriate order:

a. _____

b. _____

c. _____

d. _____

3. Analysis understanding

Scrambled order:

Apply critiquing criteria to each step of the research
Ask others to critique article, compare results
Complete comprehensive reading
Note on the article how each part of research measured up
Be familiar with critiquing criteria

Appropriate order:

a. _____

b. _____

c. _____

d. _____

e. _____

4. Synthesis understanding

Scrambled order:

Summarize study in own words
Review your own notes on the copy
Complete one handwritten 5x8 card

Appropriate order:

a. _____

b. _____

c. _____

Check your answers with those in Appendix A, Chapter 4.

ACTIVITY 4

Following are two abstracts. Respond to items 1-4 for each abstract.

1. What are the main components (variables) of the study?

2. Is the study quantitative in nature or qualitative in nature?

3. List the terms you don't know. Check their definitions in the dictionary or in the textbook.

4. Try to think like the researchers. What do you think started their interest in this topic?

Abstract 1

The incidence of chemical dependence within nursing challenges the profession to explore the phenomena of chemical dependence and its recovery. Nurses (N = 58) who were peer assistance participants were studied to examine the relationship between social support and depression. Social support was found to be significantly related to depression in this sample (r = -.642, p < .001). Over half of the sample initiated chemical use prior to completing nursing education. The findings of this study imply the need for researchers to target both practicing nurses and student nurses in future research intended to further explore chemical dependency in nursing.

Sisney, K. F. (1993). The relationship between social support and depression in recovering chemically dependent nurses. *Image: Journal of Nursing Scholarship*, 25(2), 107-112.

1. _____

_____

2. _____

3. _____

_____

4. _____

_____

Abstract 2

The presence of unreported chest pain (CP) in patients hospitalized with an acute myocardial infarction (AMI) has received only anecdotal mention in the literature, with the exception of one small study. A purposeful sample of seven informants, using an exploratory design and qualitative methods, was used to examine the experience and reporting of CP. The data indicated existence of unreported CP and represented a process of decision making in response to the symptoms associated with an AMI. The decision making process involved three stages: the experience of pain, assessing the pain, and taking action. The reporting of pain (or failure to report pain) was found to be influenced by a broad range of internal and external cues that occurred throughout the decision making process.

Schwartz, J. M. and Keller, C. (1993). Variables affecting the reporting of pain following an acute myocardial infarction. *Applied Nursing Research*, 6(1), 13-18.

1._____

_____

2._____

3._____

_____

4._____

_____

Check your answers with those in Appendix A, Chapter 4.

There is no posttest for this chapter.

REFERENCES

Schwartz, J. M. and Keller, C. (1993). Variables affecting the reporting of pain following an acute myocardial infarction. *Applied Nursing Research*, 6(1), 13-18.

Sisney, K. F. (1993). The relatonship between social support and depression in recovering chemically dependent nurses. *Image: Journal of Nursing Scholarship*, 25(2), 107-112.

5

The Literature Review

INTRODUCTION

The most common usage of the term *review of the literature* is to refer to that section of a research study in which the researcher describes the linkage between previously existing knowledge and the current study. Other research-related uses of a review of the literature are (a) developing an overall impression of what research and clinical work has been done in a given area; (b) assisting in the clarification of the research problem; (c) polishing research design ideas; and (d) finding possible data collection and data analysis strategies. This chapter aims to help you learn more about each of these uses of the literature to provide you with the basic information needed to decide whether or not a researcher has thoroughly reviewed the relevant literature and used this review to its fullest potential.

LEARNING OBJECTIVES

On completion of this chapter, the student should be able to do the following:

- Identify purposes of the literature review for research and nonresearch activities.
- Identify those paragraphs in any research study that constitute the literature review.
- Distinguish between primary and secondary sources.
- Differentiate between conceptual and data-based literature.
- Evaluate the degree to which relevant concepts and variables are discussed in the literature review.

ACTIVITY 1

What are four specific purposes of the literature review in relation to education, practice and theory development?

1. _____

2. _____

3. _____

4. _____

Check your answers with those in Appendix A, Chapter 5.

ACTIVITY 2

What is one nonresearch expected outcome of a critical review of the literature for each of the following groups? Write the correct answer next to the title on the left.

1. Clinical Nurse _____

2. Nursing Faculty _____

3. Nursing Student _____

Check your answers with those in Appendix A, Chapter 5.

ACTIVITY 3

What follows is a list of terms and examples describing either conceptual or data-based literature. Put an **A** if the example describes conceptual literature and a **B** if the example describes data-based literature. Refer to Tables 5-4 and 5-5 of the text for help.

1. _____ Scientific literature
2. _____ Theoretical literature
3. _____ Unpublished abstracts of research studies from research conferences
4. _____ Published studies in journals describing relationships between variables
5. _____ Reigel, B., Omery, A., Calvillo, E., Elsayed, N., Lee, P., Shuler, P., and Siegal, B. (1992). Moving beyond: A generative philosophy of science. *Image: Journal of Nursing Scholarship*, 24(2), 115-120
6. _____ Herr, K. and Mobily, P. (1993). Comparison of selected pain assessment tools for use with the elderly. *Applied Nursing Research*, 6(1), 39-46

Check your answers with those in Appendix A, Chapter 5.

ACTIVITY 4

Researchers who are also clinicians are interested in solving clinical problems—whether the solution is for immediate or future use. When faced with a problem in clinical practice, a clinician's common first thought is: What have others learned about this problem? The clinician usually goes first to the nursing literature to seek an answer to that question. Name five nursing journals that publish reports or research studies that you as a clinician might study to find out more about a problem.

1. _____

2. _____

3. _____

4. _____

5. _____

Check your answers with those in Appendix A, Chapter 5.

ACTIVITY 5

The review of the literature is *usually* easy to find. In the abridged version of a research report, it is clearly labeled. Most frequently, one of the early sections of the report is labeled "Review of Literature" or "Relevant Literature" or some other comparable term. It may also be separated into a literature review section and another section titled "Conceptual Framework," which presents material on the theoretical or conceptual framework which serves as the foundation for the study.

1. Examine the three articles that are in the appendices of the text. What title is given to the literature review section

   a. in Stewart Fahs and Kinney? _____

   b. in Grey, Cameron, and Thurber? _____

   c. in Hutchison and Bahr? _____

   The length of the literature review section in a journal varies. A range from two paragraphs to several paragraphs is the most common.

2. Return to the same three articles. Examine each and determine how recent the articles listed in the reference section are. They should be within 3-5 years old and should show the development of the research over time. It should read like a good detective story, in which at first there are qualitative studies which attempt to identify which variables are important to this problem or paradigm. At some point you should also see a progression as some researchers analyze each of the variables, gradually narrowing and defining the scope of the problem, while others continue to look at the problem qualitatively. Do you see this in the literature and reference section of the Stewart Fahs and Kinney article?

   Yes   No

   Write the story you see in the reference section and as described in the review of the literature.

   _____

   _____

   _____

   _____

Check your answers with those in Appendix A, Chapter 5.

ACTIVITY 6

Sometimes it is difficult to understand the distinction between primary and secondary sources of information. There is a comparison that I have always found helpful. If you are considering giving a patient an injection for pain, whose report would you feel most comfortable evaluating—the report of a family member or nurse's aide (secondary source) or the actual report of the client himself (primary source)? As a consumer of nursing research, you will also need to evaluate the credibility of research designs and reports based in part on whether they are generated from primary or secondary sources so that you know whether the information you are reading is a first-hand report or someone else's interpretation of the material.

The following words or phrases describe either primary or secondary sources. Put a **P** next to those describing primary and an **S** next to those describing secondary sources.

1. _____ Summaries of research studies
2. _____ First-hand accounts
3. _____ Biographies
4. _____ Textbooks
5. _____ Patient records
6. _____ Reports written by the researcher
7. _____ Dissertations or master's theses

Check your answers with those in Appendix A, Chapter 5.

POSTTEST

You have just completed several exercises that should have increased your ability to review critically the background literature presented in a research study. As a consumer of nursing research, you may be called on to do two very different things with research studies: critique them or summarize them. If you were asked, for instance, to review the literature in order to find an improved method for doing catheter care on your unit, you would want to perform both of these activities.

1. Which activity would you perform first? Put the number 1 next to your answer.

   _____ critique nursing research

   _____ summarize nursing research

   What is your rationale for starting with the item you chose?

   _____

   _____

2. Turn to the reference section in the Stewart Fahs and Kinney study in Appendix A of the text. Examine each of the references to determine if it is from a primary or secondary source. For each of the items below, put a **P** for primary or an **S** for secondary source.

   a. _____ Brenner, Z. R., Wood, K. M., and George, D. (1981)
   b. _____ Caprini, J. A., Zoellner, J. L., and Weisan, M. (1977)
   c. _____ Chamberlain, S. L. (1980)
   d. _____ Coley, R. M., Butler, C. D., Beck, B. I., and Mullane, J. P. (1987)
   e. _____ Gallus, A. S., Hirsh, J., Tuttle, R. J., Trebilcock, R., O'Brien, S. E., Carrol, J. J., Minden, J. H., and Hudecki, S. M. (1973)
   f. _____ Hanson, M. J. (1987)

g. _____ Hubner, C. (1986)

h. _____ Kirchhoff, K. T. (1982)

i. _____ Lundin, D. V. (1978)

j. _____ Mitchell, G. S. and Pauszek, M. E. (1987)

k. _____ Schumann, L.L., Bruya, M. A., and Henke, L. (1988)

l. _____ Sorensen, K. C. and Luckmann, J. (1986)

m. _____ VanBree, N. S., Hollerbach, A. D., and Brooks, G. P. (1984)

n. _____ Wooldridge, J. B. and Jackson, J. G. (1988)

The answers to the posttest are in the Instructor's Resource Manual. Please check with your instructor for these answers.

REFERENCES

Grey, M., Cameron, M. E., and Thurber, F. W. (1991). Coping and adaptation in children with diabetes. *Nursing Research*, 40(3), 144-149.

Herr, K. and Mobily, P. (1993). Comparision of selected pain assessment tools for use with the elderly. *Applied Nursing Research*, 6(1), 39-46.

Hutchison, C. P. and Bahr, R. T. (1991). Types and meaning of caring behaviors among elderly nursing home residents. *Image: Journal of Nursing Scholarship*, 23(2), 85-88.

Reigel, B., Omery, A., Calvillo, E., Elsayed, N., Lee, P., Shuler, P., and Siegal, B. (1992). Moving beyond: A generative philosophy of science. *Image: Journal of Nursing Scholarship*, 24(2), 115-120.

Stewart Fahs, P. S. and Kinney, M. R. (1991). The abdomen, thigh, and arm as sites for subcutaneous sodium heparin injections. *Nursing Research*, 40(4), 204-207.

CHAPTER

6

The Theoretical Framework

INTRODUCTION

For you, the critiquer, one of the most valuable aspects of the theoretical base of study is the opportunity it provides for you to see the problem through the eyes of the researcher. In developing and writing the theoretical section of a study, the researcher provides the reader with a glimpse of how he or she thinks. Our task, as critiquers, is to listen respectfully to that person's perspective and then ask ourselves the questions:

How clearly do I understand the researcher's argument?
Did the theoretical framework connect all the pieces of the study?

Most of the exercises in this chapter address the first question. Your ability to answer the second question will improve as you complete the course for which these books are the text.

LEARNING OBJECTIVES

On completion of this chapter, the student should be able to do the following:

- Discuss the importance of the following terms to a piece of research:
  a. concept
  b. theoretical framework or theoretical rationale
  c. conceptual definition
  d. operational definition
- Identify the major concepts in a given study.
- Evaluate the relationship of a given theoretical framework to the relevant study and to clinical practice.
- Distinguish between a conceptual definition and an operational definition.
- Determine which of the phenomena central to nursing is addressed in specific studies.

ACTIVITY 1

1. Define, in your own words, the following terms:

Concept _____

Theoretical framework _____

Conceptual definition _____

Operational definition _____

2. Following are excerpts from some studies. Determine whether the excerpt is an example of a concept, a theoretical framework, a conceptual definition, or an operational definition.

   a. person as an adaptive system

   _____

   b. Cultural care is the "subjectively and objectively learned and transmitted values, beliefs and patterned lifeways that assist, support, facilitate, or enable another individual or group to maintain their well-being, health, to improve their human condition and lifeway, or to deal with illness, handicaps or death."

   _____

   c. . . . afterdrop, the fall in core temperature following completion of cardiac surgery, . . .

   _____

   d. "Selection of study variables was guided by the Roy Adaptation Model of Nursing (Roy and Andrews, 1991) and the findings from research on responses to cesarean birth. The Roy Adaptation Model depicts the individual as an adaptive system who interacts with constantly changing environmental stimuli. Four modes of adaptation are taken into account: physiological, self-concept, role function, and interdependence." (Fawcett, et al., 1993)

   _____

   e. "Ongoing recovery was . . . the number of months a subject was a peer assistance program participant without having experienced more than one relapse. Relapse was . . . testing positive for drugs and/or alcohol in response to a random urinalysis drug screen." (Sisney, 1993)

   _____

Check your answers with those in Appendix A, Chapter 6.

ACTIVITY 2

As explained in the text, concepts are the building blocks of a study. As you strengthen your ability to recognize the critical concepts in a study, you will be able to follow more easily and more quickly the researcher's thinking from concept to variable to hypothesis to instruments to outcomes.

Identify the major concepts in each of the following statements of purpose:

1. This study was designed to assess factors associated with afterdrop, . . . and determine the validity of noninvasive measures of temperature to predict core temperature in the severely hypothermic patient. (Heidenreich, Giuffre, Doorley, 1992)

   _____   _____

   _____   _____

2. The relationships among uncertainty, hope, symptom severity, control preference, and psychosocial adjustment were examined in persons having radiotherapy for cancer. (Christman, 1990)

   _____   _____

   _____   _____

   _____   _____

3. The effects of cesarean birth information given in childbirth preparation classes on maternal postpartum reaction to unplanned cesarean delivery were examined. (Fawcett, Pollio, Tully, Baron, Henklein, Jones, 1993)

   _____

   _____

4. This pilot study was designed to describe heart rate variability (HRV), anxiety, anger, denial, and depression during the first four days and six months after acute myocardial infarction (AMI). (Buchanan, Cowan, Burr, Waldron, and Kogan, 1993)

   _____   _____

   _____   _____

   _____   _____

5. Body image, as a component of self-concept, was compared in four groups of women (N = 257) who received the most common types of treatment for breast cancer: mastectomy, mastectomy with delayed reconstruction, mastectomy with immediate reconstruction, and conservative surgery. (Mock, 1993)

   _____   _____

   _____

Check your answers with those in Appendix A, Chapter 6.

ACTIVITY 3

Before turning to the actual critiquing of the theoretical aspects of a particular study, practice with one more bit of information may be helpful. One needs to be able to distinguish between a conceptual and an operational definition. At times this is easier said than done.

Let's take the word *smoking*. Conceptually (with the help of a dictionary), smoking is defined as follows: "to inhale and exhale the fumes of burning plant material, and especially tobacco" (*Webster's New Collegiate Dictionary*, p.1097). A researcher is interested in the effects of different levels of smoking upon fetal growth and development. *Heavy smoking* is one level of this independent variable. But how much smoking is necessary to be labeled as "heavy smoking"? One pack of cigarettes per day? Per week? Two packs? More? Less? Cigarettes only? Twenty cigarettes to the box or pack? Twenty-four? One example of an operational definition of the term *heavy smoking* is the following:

Heavy smokers are women between the ages of 18 and 40 years of age who smoke more than two packs of cigarettes per day with tar and nicotine levels greater than 7 mg and 0.5 mg respectively.

Remember, an operational definition should be so clear that you, the reader, can picture it in your mind.

Now try your hand at spotting operational definitions. Which of the following are operational definitions?

1. _____ A mentally retarded person is anyone with diminished intellectual abilities.

2. _____ Height will be determined by measuring the distance between two lines. The lines are determined by laying the child on a piece of paper and then marking the level of the crown of the head and the heel of the right leg.

3. _____ Level of occupation is categorized according to Roe's Two-Way Classification of Occupation (Row, 1956).

4. _____ Personality is defined as having three facets: dynamic traits, ability traits, and temperament traits.

5. _____ A moderate level of anxiety is indicated by a score of 45 on the State Anxiety Scale.

Check your answers with those in Appendix A, Chapter 6.

ACTIVITY 4

1. Name the four central phenomena of interest in nursing theory.

   a. _____

   b. _____

   c. _____

   d. _____

2. Following are several statements describing theoretical frameworks used in specific studies (some of the researchers use the term "conceptual framework" but for the purpose of this activity assume that conceptual or theoretical are synonymous). Put a **B** next to those studies using theory borrowed from other disciplines and an **N** next to those using one or more of the phenomena found in nursing theories.

   a. _____ "The conceptual framework for this study unified the concepts of social distance and appraisal to investigate interrelationships in caregiving." (Sayles-Cross, 1993)

   b. _____ "The Roy Adaptation Model depicts the individual as an adaptive system who interacts with constantly changing environmental stimuli. Four modes of adaptation are taken into account: physiological, self-concept, role function, and interdependence. Nursing intervention involves increasing, decreasing, maintaining, removing, or otherwise altering or changing relevant focal and/or contextual environmental stimuli. In the present study, the contextual stimulus was a nursing intervention, operationalized as the experimental and control treatment childbirth preparation classes. . . . " (Fawcett, et al., 1993)

   c. _____ "This study examines the relationship of self-esteem and social support to problem-focused coping behavior of 101 individuals with multiple sclerosis, a chronic progressive disease." (O'Brien, 1993)

   d. _____ "The effects of cognitive-behavioral group therapy, focused visual imagery group therapy, and education-discussion groups on cognition, depression, hopelessness and dissatisfaction with life were studied among depressed nursing home residents." (Abraham, Neundorfer, and Currie, 1992)

   e. _____ "In an effort to relate the potentially multiple determinants of children's positive health behaviors systematically, the Interaction Model of Client Health Behavior (IMCHB) (Cox, 1982) was selected as the conceptual framework to direct the study. . . . The model is nursing based, client focused, and holistic because it considers clients and their unique characteristics, along with factors external to the client, as relevant in explaining health behavior."

   f. _____ "Hutchinson (1987) has reported that positive self-care outcomes may be directly linked to job satisfaction. Thus it is postulated that the exercise of self-care agency, described by Oren (1985) as the process of acting in one's own behalf to maintain personal well-being, could be one internal coping mechanism used by nurses . . . ." (Behm and Frank, 1992)

3. After you have checked your answers with those in Appendix A, reread the items in #2 of Activity 4. Which of the four phenomena central to nursing theory is being addressed in those items identified as being based in nursing theory?

a. _____

b. _____

c. _____

Check your answers with those in Appendix A, Chapter 6.

ACTIVITY 5

You have dissected several components of that part of a research study known as the theoretical framework. You now need to assess the quality of that section of the research report. Review the critiquing questions found in Chapter 6 of the text.

Use the grid that follows and critique the theoretical framework portion of the three studies found in the appendices of the text, i.e., Stewart Fahs and Kinney; Grey, Cameron, and Thurber; and Hutchison and Bahr.

In the grid, put **F** if the Stewart Fahs and Kinney study satisfied that particular criterion; put **G** if the Grey, Cameron, and Thurber study did; and put **H** if the Hutchison and Bahr study did.

Look over the grid. Which study received the highest marks, i.e., met the greatest number of criteria? Did any study meet all of the criteria? A mark on either the "Well Done" or "OK" box would qualify a study for meeting that criterion. Be surprised if one of the studies meets every criterion. It is extremely difficult to do.

1. Which study is the strongest in terms of its theoretical base?

_____

_____

2. How does this information influence your thinking about this particular study?

_____

_____

_____

CRITIQUING GRID

	Well Done	OK	Needs Help	Not Applicable
1. If clearly identified— Could I find it?				
2. Concepts a. conceptual definition(s) found				
b. conceptual definition(s) clear				
c. operational definition(s) found				
d. operational definition(s) clear				
3. Satisfied with operational definitions of conceptual definitions				
4. Enough literature reviewed a. for an expert in the area				
b. for a nurse with some knowledge				
c. for a nurse reading outside of area of specialty or interest				
5. Thinking of researcher can be followed through theoretical material to hypotheses or questions				
6. Relationships among propositions stated———clearly stated				
7. Use of concepts is consistent from beginning to end				
8. Theory a. borrowed				
b. findings related to nursing				
9. Findings related back to theoretical base, can find each concept from the theoretical section discussed in the "Results" section of the report				

Check your answers with those in Appendix A, Chapter 6.

POSTTEST

Put a **T** (for True) or an **F** (for false) in front of the following statements. Once you have determined that an item is false, correct it so that it becomes a true statement.

1. _____ The following phrases are synonymous:
   a. theoretical rationale
   b. theoretical framework
   c. conceptual framework
   d. operational definitions

2. _____ The theoretical framework of a study lays the foundation for the entire study including the design and methodology.

3. _____ Nursing no longer needs to borrow theoretical constructs from other disciplines; it has its own theories from which to work.

4. _____ The section of the report titled "Review of the Literature" is the most likely place to find the theoretical rationale of the study.

5. List the four phenomena central to the development of nursing theory.

   a. _____

   b. _____

   c. _____

   d. _____

6. Identify the operational definitions in the following list:

   a. Assertiveness is defined as the ability to express oneself clearly and distinctly in situations with varying degrees of personal threat.

   b. Successful housebreaking of a puppy is:
   - no evidence of urine or feces in the house for 7 consecutive days
   - puppy goes to door and barks to be let out

   c. A student in good standing in the School of Nursing meets the following criteria:
   - maintains a 2.00 GPA (on a four-point scale) with a minimum grade of C in each prerequisite and major course
   - maintains steady progress toward the completion of the degree

   d. Fever is present when the oral temperature using a mercury thermometer reaches 38.2 degrees Celsius.

In each of the following research briefs, identify the concepts you would expect to find discussed in the theoretical section of the research report.

7. A longitudinal study of 105 couples . . . addresses whether there is a change in marital satisfaction throughout the perinatal period and whether any changes in the marriage or the labor and delivery might be attributable to the type of preparation for childbirth engaged in by the couple. (Moore, 1983)

_____

_____

_____

8. Recent research findings contradict the notion that premenstrual and menstrual symptoms constitute two mutually exclusive categories of perimenstrual distress. The purposes of this study were to describe the prevalence of distress associated with menstruation in a community population and to determine whether perimenstrual distress could be regarded as a single construct. (Woods, 1982)

_____

_____

_____

9. Relationships among sources of social support and criterion measures of functioning of single parents were examined. (Norbeck and Scheiner, 1982)

_____

_____

_____

10. What are the effects of two types of information (sensation or procedure oriented) about an impending threatening event (barium enema) on subjects' expectations and the intensity of their emotional response to the event? (Hartfield, Cason, and Cason, 1982)

_____

_____

_____

11. List three reasons supporting the importance of the theoretical rationale of a study.

a. _____

b. _____

c. _____

The answers to the posttest are in the Instructor's Resource Manual. Please check with your instructor for these answers.

REFERENCES

Abraham, I. L., Neundorfer, M. M., and Currie, L. J. (1992). Effects of groups interventions on cognition and depression in nursing home residents. *Nursing Research*, 41(4), 196-202.

Behm, L. K. and Fran, D. I. (1992). The relationship between self-care agency and job satisfaction in public health nurses. *Applied Nursing Research*, 5(1), 28-29.

Buchanan, L. M., Cowan, M., Burr, R., Waldron, C., and Kogan, H. (1993). Measurement of recovery from myocardial infarction using heart rate variablility. *Nursing Research*, 42(2), 74-78.

Christman, N. J. (1990). Uncertainty and adjustment during radiotherapy. *Nursing Research*, 39(1), 17-20.

Farrand, L. L. and Cox, C. L. (1993). Determinants of positive health behavior in middle childhood. *Nursing Research*, 42(4), 208-213.

Fawcett, J., Pollio, N., Tully, A., Baron, M., Henklein, J. C., and Jones, R. C. (1993). Effects of information on adaption to cesarean birth. *Nursing Research*, 42(1), 49-53.

Heidenreich, T., Giuffre, M., and Doorley, J. (1992). Temperature and temperature measurement after induced hypothermia. *Nursing Research*, 41(5), 296-300.

Mock, V. (1993). Body image in women treated for breast cancer. *Nursing Research*, 42(3), 153-157.

Moore, D. (1983). Prepared childbirth and marital satisfaction during the antepartum and postpartum periods. *Nursing Research*, 32(2), 73-79.

Norbeck, J. S. and Sheiner, M. (1982). Sources of social support related to single-parent functioning. *Research in Nursing and Health*, 5(1), 3-12.

O'Brien, M. T. (1993). Multiple sclerosis: The relationship among self-esteem, social support, and coping behavior. *Applied Nursing Research*, 6(2), 54-63.

Sayles-Cross, S. Perceptions of familial caregivers of elder adults. *Image: Journal of Nursing Scholarship*, 25(2), 88-92.

Sisney, K. F. (1993). The relationship between social support and depression in recovering chemically dependent nurses. *Image: Journal of Nursing Scholarship*, 25(2), 107-112.

Woods, N. F., Most, A., and Dery, G. K. (1982). Toward a construct of perimenstrual distress. *Research in Nursing and Health*, 5(3), 123-136.

7

The Problem Statement and Hypothesis

INTRODUCTION

This chapter focuses on the problem statement and hypothesis. If done correctly, a problem statement can be very helpful to you as a consumer of nursing research because it very concisely—usually in one or two sentences—describes the essence of the research study. For the nurse who is considering the results of a given study in daily practice, the two primary concerns are (a) locate the problem statement, and (b) critique it. The hypothesis or the research question provides the most succinct link between the underlying theoretical base and the research design. Thus its analysis is pivotal to the analysis of the entire research study.

LEARNING OBJECTIVES

On completion of this chapter, the student should be able to do the following:

- Identify terms related to problem statement and hypotheses.
- Differentiate between a "good" problem statement and a problem statement with limitations.
- Distinguish between each of the following:
  a. research hypothesis
  b. statistical hypothesis
  c. research question
  d. directional hypothesis
  e. nondirectional hypothesis
- Distinguish between independent and dependent variables.

ACTIVITY 1

Match the term in Column B with the appropriate phrase in Column A. Not all terms from Column B will be used.

Column A

1. _____ an interrogative sentence or declarative statement about the relationship between two or more variables

2. _____ the variable that has the presumed effect on the second variable

3. _____ the variable that is not manipulated

Column B

a. testability
b. independent variable
c. variables
d. dependent variable
e. problem statement
f. hypothesis

4. _____ a property of the problem that indicates it is
measurable by either qualitative or quantitative
methods

5. _____ the concepts or properties that are operationalized
and studied

Check your answers with those in Appendix A, Chapter 7.

ACTIVITY 2

A good problem statement exhibits four criteria. Read the problem statements below and examine them to determine if each of the four criteria is present. Following each problem statement is a list representing the four criteria (a-d). Circle yes or no to indicate whether each criterion is met.

The problem statement:

a. clearly and unambiguously identifies the variables under consideration.
b. clearly expresses the variables' relationship to each other.
c. specifies the nature of the population being studied.
d. implies the possibility of empirical testing.

1. The purpose of this study was to examine the paid work role as a critical factor and determinant of health risk of older widows during their conjugal bereavement. (Aber, 1992)

   Criterion a: Yes No
   Criterion b: Yes No
   Criterion c: Yes No
   Criterion d: Yes No

2. The present study compared the effects of thermal biofeedback combined with progressive muscle relaxation and progressive muscle relaxation alone in the reduction of blood pressures. (Bok Ha, Ja Ro, Hiang Song, Cho Kim, Seung Kim, Sook Yoo, 1993)

   Criterion a: Yes No
   Criterion b: Yes No
   Criterion c: Yes No
   Criterion d: Yes No

3. In particular, the relationship between social support and depression in a convenience sample of 58 chemically dependent subjects who were participants in a state legislated peer assistance program for nurses and were, consequently, involved in the ongoing process of recovery was explored. (Sisney, 1993)

   Criterion a: Yes No
   Criterion b: Yes No
   Criterion c: Yes No
   Criterion d: Yes No

Check your answers with those in Appendix A, Chapter 7.

ACTIVITY 3

The ability to distinguish between independent and dependent variables is a crucial preliminary step to determine whether or not a given research hypothesis is a succinct statement of the relationship between two variables. Identify the variables in the following examples. Decide which is the independent (presumed cause) variable and which is the dependent (presumed effect) variable.

1. The use of cathode ray terminals (CRTs) increases the incidence of birth defects.

    Independent variable _____

    Dependent variable _____

2. Individuals with birth defects have a higher incidence of independence/dependence conflict than individuals without birth defects.

    Independent variable _____

    Dependent variable _____

3. What is the relationship between daily moderate consumption of white wine and serum cholesterol levels?

    Independent variable _____

    Dependent variable _____

4. Problem-oriented recording leads to more effective patient care than narrative recording.

    Independent variable _____

    Dependent variable _____

5. Nurses and physicians differ in the way they view the extended-role concept for nurses.

    Independent variable _____

    Dependent variable _____

Check your answers with those in Appendix A, Chapter 7.

ACTIVITY 4

Now take each hypothesis (or research question) from Activity 3 and label it with the appropriate abbreviation from the key provided. More than one abbreviation from the key may be used to describe each item.

KEY: RQ = research question
DH = directional hypothesis
NDH = nondirectional hypothesis
H_R = research hypothesis
H_O = statistical hypothesis

1. _____ The use of cathode ray terminals (CRTs) increases the incidence of birth defects.

2. _____ Individuals with birth defects have a higher incidence of independence /dependence conflicts than individuals without birth defects.

3. _____ What is the relationship between daily moderate consumption of white wine and serum cholesterol levels?

4. _____ Problem-oriented recording leads to more effective patient care than narrative recording.

5. _____ Nurses and physicians differ in the way they view the extended-role concept for nurses.

Check your answers with those in Appendix A, Chapter 7.

ACTIVITY 5

The next step is to practice writing hypotheses of different types. Return to the five hypotheses you labeled in Activity 4. Each was labeled as a specific type of hypothesis or research question. Rewrite each hypothesis to meet the conditions of the remaining four types of questions or hypotheses. The first problem is partially completed to provide an example.

1. DH   The use of CRTs increases the incidence of birth defects.

   NDH   The use of CRTs influences the incidence of birth defects.

   H_R The use of CRTs increases the incidence of birth defects.

   RQ   _____

   H_O _____

2. DH   _____

   NDH   _____

   H_R _____

RQ _____

H_O _____

3. DH _____

NDH _____

H_R _____

RQ _____

H_O _____

4. DH _____

NDH _____

H_R _____

RQ _____

H_O _____

5. DH _____

NDH _____

H_R _____

RQ _____

H_O _____

Check your answers with those in Appendix A, Chapter 7.

POSTTEST

1. Review the Stewart Fahs and Kinney (1991) article in Appendix A of the text.

   a. Highlight the problem statement.

   b. List the independent variable(s). _____

   c. List the dependent variable(s). _____

   d. Evaluate the problem statement in the Stewart Fahs and Kinney article in terms of the four criteria listed below.

Criterion a: clearly and unambiguously identifies the variables under consideration
  Yes   No

Criterion b: clearly expresses the variables' relationship to each other
  Yes   No

Criterion c: specifies the nature of the population being studied
  Yes   No

Criterion d: implies the possibility of empirical testing
  Yes   No

2. Choose the terms from the key provided that best describe items a-h. Write the appropriate abbreviation in the space provided. More than one abbreviation from the key may be used to describe each item.

   KEY: RQ = research question
         DH = directional hypothesis
         NDH = nondirectional hypothesis
         H_R = research hypothesis
         H_O = statistical hypothesis

   a. _____ There will be no change in self-rated body image among women in the three patient groups.
   b. _____ What is the relationship between organizational climate dimensions and job satisfaction of nurses in neonatal intensive care units?
   c. _____ The higher the perceived parental support, the lower the girls' general fearfulness.
   d. _____ There will be a significant difference in pre-post changes in cognitive development level between undergraduate nursing students who have completed a research course and those who have not.
   e. _____ The posttest mean of selected psychological variables for the experimental group will be lower than that of the control group.
   f. _____ There will be no association found between the level of social support and self-care health practices.
   g. _____ The educational preparation of a nurse (e.g., AA, diploma, BS) will affect his/her ability to conduct thorough patient interviews.
   h. _____ What is the level of postoperative infection following the use of clean tracheotomy care?

3. Fill in the blanks in the following sentences with the appropriate word or words from the list provided. Not all the words in the list will be used.

research hypothesis	null hypothesis
predicts	validity
statistical hypothesis	directional hypothesis
testing	declarative statement
nondirectional hypothesis	research question

a. The hypothesis is a vehicle for _____ the

_____ of the assumptions of the theoretical framework
of a research study.

b. A hypothesis transposes the question posed by the research problem into a

_____ _____ that

_____ the relationship between two or more variables.

c. _____ hypotheses are more common than

_____ hypotheses in studies that utilize deductive
reasoning.

d. A _____ hypothesis is also known as the

_____ hypothesis.

4. Assume that the information in the following vignette is accurate and well supported by
   previous research. Write a directional research hypothesis, a nondirectional research
   hypothesis, a null hypothesis, and a research question.

   During the first week of the semester at Commuter College a student can add or drop
   classes without penalty. Approximately 50% of the students plan to add or drop one class
   during this first week of class. Add/drops require the signature of the instructor of the
   class. The consequences of this requirement are (a) people stand in line outside most
   classrooms; (b) parking garages open at 7 a.m. and fill very quickly; and (c) traffic moves
   very slowly from the freeway to campus. Better movement of the traffic and ease in
   parking are two concerns of the campus administration.

   a. Nondirectional research hypothesis _____

   _____

   _____

   b. Directional research hypothesis _____

   _____

   _____

c. Statistical (null) hypothesis (Hint: This will be easier to write if you tie it to one of the

already written research hypotheses.) _____

_____

_____

d. Research question

_____

_____

The answers to the posttest are in the Instructor's Resource Manual. Please check with your instructor for these answers.

REFERENCES

Aber, C. (1992). Spousal death, a threat to women's health: Paid work as a "Resistance Resource." *Image: Journal of Nursing Scholarship*, 24(2), 95-100.

Bok Ha, Ja Ro, Hiang Song, Cho Kim, Seung Kim, Sook Yoo (1993). The effect of thermal biofeedback and progressive muscle relaxation training in reducing blood pressure of patients with essential hypertension. *Image: Journal of Nursing Scholarship*, 25(3), 204-207.

Sisney, K. F. (1993). The relationship between social support and depression in recovering chemically dependent nurses. *Image: Journal of Nursing Scholarship*, 25(2), 107-112.

CHAPTER

8

Introduction to Design

INTRODUCTION

The term *research design* is used to describe the overall plan of a particular study. The design is the researcher's plan for answering specific research questions in the most accurate and efficient way possible. The design ties together the present research problem, the knowledge of the past, and the implications for the future. Thus the choice of a design reflects the researcher's experience, expertise, knowledge, and biases.

LEARNING OBJECTIVES

On completion of this chapter, the student should be able to do the following:

- Identify the major components of a research design.
- Appropriately use specified terms relevant to research design.
- Identify threats to internal validity.
- Identify threats to external validity.
- State the relationship between the research design and internal and external validity.
- Critically analyze the strengths and limitations of the chosen design for a specific study.

ACTIVITY 1

The term *research design* is an all-encompassing term for the overall plan to answer the research questions, including the method and specific plans to control other factors which could influence the results of the study.

1. In order to become acquainted with the major elements in the design of a study, read the study on subcutaneous heparin injection sites by Stewart Fahs and Kinney in Appendix A in the text and answer the six questions that follow.

   a. What was the setting of the study?

   _____

   b. Who were the subjects?

   _____

c. How many persons were in the sample?

_____

d. How was the sample selected?

_____

e. How were events measured?

_____

f. Were any of these elements missing?

_____

If your answer is yes, what effect do you think this would have on your understanding of the study and eventually your incorporation of the results in your practice?

_____

_____

Check your answers with those in Appendix A, Chapter 8.

ACTIVITY 2

Listed below are some terms that are relevant to the topic of research design. Refer to Chapter 8 of the text or other reference material to develop a working definition of each term. A "working definition" is a definition in your own words that you understand, not a definition copied directly from the book.

1. Research design _____

_____

2. Accuracy _____

_____

3. Control _____

_____

4. Feasibility _____

_____

5. Homogeneous sampling _____

_____

6. Random sampling _____

_____

7. Internal validity _____

_____

8. External validity _____

_____

Check your answers with those in Appendix A, Chapter 8.

ACTIVITY 3

For each of the following situations identify the type of threat to internal validity and how you could correct for this threat.

1. Nurses on a maternity unit want to study the effect of a hospital-based teaching program on mothers' confidence in caring for their infants. They mail out a survey one month after discharge.

_____

2. In a study of the results of a hypertension teaching program conducted at a senior center, the blood pressures taken by volunteers using their personal equipment were compared before and after the program.

_____

3. A major increase in cigarette taxes occurs during a one-year follow-up study of the impact of a smoking cessation program.

_____

4. The smoking cessation rates of an experimental group consisting of volunteers for a smoking cessation program with daily meetings were compared with the results of a control group of persons who wanted to quit on their own without a special program.

_____

5. Although 30% of the subjects dropped out of a study of employment after a job training program for homeless families, 90% of the persons completing the program were

employed within two months and the program was deemed successful for all homeless families. Ninety percent of the dropouts were single women with at least two preschool children.

_____

6. The researcher measured the confidence and accuracy of nursing students in calculating drug dosage and solutions at the beginning, middle, and end of a two-week course using a standardized calculation exam.

_____

Check your answers with those in Appendix A, Chapter 8.

ACTIVITY 4

Read each of the following situations. After you have read the situation, rate the study as to the degree of internal validity and external validity by placing an X on the scale provided. (Note that +++ indicates high validity and --- indicates low validity.) Provide a brief rationale for each of your ratings.

Situation 1: Conduct a new preoperative teaching program for patients admitted for surgery. Measure the level of anxiety in each patient one hour before surgery. Conclude that low anxiety is the result of the new teaching program and recommend its widespread use.

Internal validity: ---   -/+   +++

Rationale _____

_____

_____

_____

External validity: ---   -/+   +++

Rationale _____

_____

_____

_____

Situation 2: To test the effectiveness of a comprehensive health care program for first-time adolescent mothers and their infants, 243 mother-infant pairs were randomly assigned to one of two groups. The control group received routine well-baby care. The experimental group received routine care plus a comprehensive follow-up program, health teaching, and discussion of return to school and family planning information. The results for the experimental group were lower repeat pregnancy rates, infants more likely to be fully immunized at 12 months, higher continuation of clinic visits, and lower use of the emergency room than the control group. There was no difference in rate of return to school. (From O'Sullivan, A. L. and Jacobsen, B. S. [1992]. A randomized trial of a health care program for first-time adolescent mothers and their infants. *Nursing Research*, 41, 210-215.)

Internal validity: ---   -/+   +++

Rationale _____

_____

_____

_____

External validity: ---   -/+   +++

Rationale _____

_____

_____

_____

Check your answers with those in Appendix A, Chapter 8.

ACTIVITY 5

Use the critiquing criteria found in Chapter 8 to critique the design of the study of heparin injections by Stewart Fahs and Kinney found in the appendix of the text.

_____

_____

_____

_____

_____

Check your answers with those in Appendix A, Chapter 8.

POSTTEST

1. What are the major components included when discussing the design of a study?

   a. _____

   b. _____

   c. _____

   d. _____

   e. _____

2. Match the term in Column B with the appropriate phrase in Column A. Not all terms from Column B will be used.

   Column A   Column B

   1. _____ a term that indicates how well a study   a. control
            is put together to control rival explanations   b. selection bias
   2. _____ holding constant the conditions of the study   c. reliability-
   3. _____ all aspects of a study logically follow from   d. maturation
            the problem statement   e. internal validity
   4. _____ the believability between this study and the   f. external validity
            world at large   g. accuracy
   5. _____ the developmental, biological or psychological   h. history
            processes that operate within a person over a time

The answers to the posttest are in the Instructor's Resource Manual. Please check with your instructor for these answers.

REFERENCE

O'Sullivan, A. L. and Jacobsen, B. S. (1992). A randomized trial of a health care program for first-time adolescent mothers and their infants. *Nursing Research*, 41, 210-215.

9

Experimental and Quasi-experimental Design

INTRODUCTION

This chapter contains exercises for only two categories of design: experimental and quasi-experimental. These types of designs allow researchers to test the effects of nursing actions and make statements about cause-effect relationships. Therefore, they can be very helpful in testing solutions to nursing practice problems. However, a researcher chooses the design that allows a given situation or problem to be studied in the most accurate and effective way possible. Thus, not all problems are amenable to immediate study by these two types of designs. Rather, the choice of design is dependent on the development of research relevant to the problem plus the researcher's knowledge, experience, expertise, resources, and biases.

LEARNING OBJECTIVES

On completion of this chapter, the student should be able to do the following:

• Identify experimental and quasi-experimental categories of research design.
• Compare and contrast experimental and quasi-experimental research designs.
• Critique the type of design used in specific studies.
• Critique the application potential of the findings of specific experimental and quasi-experimental studies.

ACTIVITY 1

O'Sullivan and Jacobsen conducted a study of the effectiveness of a health care follow-up program for adolescent mothers. They randomly assigned 243 mother-infant pairs to one of two groups. One group received routine well-baby care. The other group received routine care plus extensive follow-up care. After 12 months they found that the group receiving follow-up care had fewer repeat pregnancies, infants were more likely to be more fully immunized, and they used the emergency room less than the group receiving only routine care. (O'Sullivan, A. L. and Jacobsen, B. S. [1992]. A randomized trial of a health care program for first-time adolescent mothers and their infants. *Nursing Research*, 41, 210-215.)

1. The classic experiment has three properties: randomization, control, and manipulation. How were each of these conditions applied in this study and why was this done?

a. Randomization _____

_____

b. Control _____

_____

c. Manipulation _____

_____

2. How does this study handle potential threats to internal validity, such as maturation, history, or selection?

_____

_____

3. List the implications of this study for nursing practice.

_____

_____

4. What difference would there be in interpreting the results if the researcher had not used randomization?

_____

_____

5. What difference would there be in interpreting the results if the researcher had not used a control group?

_____

_____

Check your answers with those in Appendix A, Chapter 9.

ACTIVITY 2

The inservice education department wants to test a program to educate and change nurses' attitudes in a positive direction toward the chemically dependent nurse. They have a questionnaire which measures nurses' information and attitudes toward chemically dependent nurses. They also have a teaching plan that will provide information on the disease concept of chemical dependency, treatment options, and recovering nurses who will tell their story to the class. Your responsibility is to design a study to measure the outcome of this intervention program.

1. Write a plan for a Solomon four-group design.

_____

_____

_____

_____

2. Assume you need 30 nurses for each group. How would you assign nurses to each group?

_____

_____

_____

3. What would you do to the first two groups for a pretest?

_____

_____

4. How would you do the experimental treatment?

_____

_____

5. Based on your reading, for what types of issues is this design particularly effective?

_____

_____

6. What is the major advantage of this type of design?

_____

_____

Check your answers with those in Appendix A, Chapter 9.

ACTIVITY 3

A researcher wanted to test the effects of a postoperative teaching intervention program, but the patients were too ill to complete pretests before the intervention was conducted. By random assignment, patients were placed either into a control group who received routine postoperative care or into an experimental group who received an experimental teaching program. At the time of discharge it was found that patients in the experimental group had more knowledge and less anxiety about postoperative care than the patients receiving routine care.

1. How did the researcher control for bias in the study?

   _____

2. What are some of the possible reasons the researcher used this type of design? What are some of the advantages?

   _____

   _____

   _____

Check your answers with those in Appendix A, Chapter 9.

ACTIVITY 4

A registered nurse is working at a clinic that provides free blood pressure measurements two days a week, Monday and Thursday. On the first Monday and Thursday of the month the research RN measures blood pressures for all the people who appear and asks them to participate in a six-week study. As part of the study, she invites the Thursday clients to stay for a class covering such topics as stress reduction, diet, and hypertensive medication regimes.

At the conclusion of the six weeks of classes, all 25 Monday clients and 25 Thursday clients have their blood pressures taken, and the nurse analyzes the results. She finds there is a statistically significant drop from the mean pretest blood pressure readings and the mean posttest readings of the experimental (Thursday) group only.

1. The nurse researcher concludes that the class is directly responsible for the drop in blood pressure. Do you agree? Why or why not?

   _____

2. Can you think of at least three other explanations that could account for the drop in blood pressure of the experimental group?

   _____

   _____

3. Do you think the design of this study would provide you with enough data, based only on the information in the situation, that you would be willing to change your practice based on the results? Why or why not, from a design perspective?

_____

_____

_____

Check your answers with those in Appendix A, Chapter 9.

ACTIVITY 5

An experimental case management program was implemented on a surgical unit of a hospital. A second surgical unit with similar patient composition but no case management program served as a control unit. Patients from both units completed patient satisfaction questionnaires prior to discharge.

1. Critique this study from a design perspective.

_____

_____

2. Assume that the findings of this study indicate greater patient satisfaction on the case management unit. Based solely on the results of this study, will you recommend that your unit adopt case management?

_____

_____

Check your answers with those in Appendix A, Chapter 9.

ACTIVITY 6

All members of a group of people with newly diagnosed hypertension had their blood pressures taken at the beginning of a series of classes. None of the participants had previous classes on management of hypertension. They are given an eight-week series of classes on low sodium diets, weight loss, and stress reduction. At the end of eight weeks, all members of the group had their blood pressure taken. There was a statistically significant drop in blood pressure from levels prior to the classes.

1. From your general knowledge as a nurse, what do you think caused this drop?

_____

_____

2. Do you think it is possible, based on the information generated by this one group, to state a clear cause-effect relationship based on this study?

_____

_____

3. What type of study or studies would you like to have conducted before you would be willing to change what you teach patients about hypertension?

_____

_____

Check your answers with those in Appendix A, Chapter 9.

ACTIVITY 7

A study was conducted to evaluate the effect of soothing music on blood pressure recordings in a group of volunteers. Blood pressures recordings were taken prior to music being played, at two-minute intervals while the music played for 10 minutes, and then after the music was turned off. It was found that each subject's blood pressure was slightly lower when the music was played than before or after.

1. How do you think the data generated by this study could be of clinical value to you as a practitioner?

_____

_____

2. Is there any additional information that you would like about this study from a design perspective?

_____

_____

Check your answers with those in Appendix A, Chapter 9.

ACTIVITY 8

You may be questioning why anyone would use a quasi-experimental design if an experimental design has the advantage of being so much stronger and enables the researcher to generalize the results to a wider population. In what instances might it be necessary to use a quasi-experimental design?

_____

_____

_____

Check your answers with those in Appendix A, Chapter 9.

POSTTEST

1. Identify whether the following studies are experimental or quasi-experimental. Use the abbreviations from the key provided.

   KEY: E = experimental

          Q = quasi-experimental

   a. _____ From two groups of randomly chosen post-operative clients, one group is randomly assigned a new dressing-change technique, and the incidence of post-operative infection is observed.

   b. _____ Patients on two separate units are given a patient satisfaction test. Then patients on one unit receive care from the same nurse for four days, while the patients on the other unit receive care from the usual rotation of nurses. At the end of four days the satisfaction test is repeated on both units.

   c. _____ Students are randomly assigned to two groups. One is a new teaching program and the other the usual classroom teaching. Both groups receive the same posttest to evaluate learning.

   d. _____ A group of postoperative patients are contacted one week after hospital discharge to evaluate the outcome of a discharge teaching program.

2. Identify the type of experimental or quasi-experimental design for each of the following examples. Use the numbers from the key provided.

   KEY: 1 = One group pretest-posttest

          2 = True experiment

          3 = Nonequivalent control group

          4 = Time series

          5 = After only experiment

          6 = After only nonequivalent control group

          7 = Solomon four-group

   a. _____ Blood pressure and pulse rates are monitored every five minutes before, during, and after an exercise program.

   b. _____ Nurses are randomly assigned to a new self-study program or to the usual EKG program. Knowledge of EKGs is tested before and after the program for both groups.

c. _____ Babies who tested positive on toxicology screening at birth are randomly assigned into groups to either receive routine care or to receive a special public health nurse intervention program. Health outcomes are tested at six months.

d. _____ School nurse clinic is set up at one school. Health care outcomes from that school are measured and compared with health outcomes at a comparable school without a clinic.

e. _____ An employment satisfaction survey was conducted in a hospital before and after implementation of a new nurse management system.

f. _____ Diabetic patients were randomly assigned to either one of two control groups receiving routine home health care or to one of two groups with a new diabetic teaching program. Patients in one of the control groups and in one of the teaching groups took a test of diabetic knowledge as soon as they were assigned to a group; patients in the other two groups were not pretested. All patients completed a posttest at the conclusion of the three-week program.

g. _____ A new peer AIDS prevention program was implemented in one high school. A second high school without the program served as a control group. An AIDS knowledge test was administered at both schools before and after the program was completed.

The answers to the posttest are in the Instructor's Resource Manual. Please check with your instructor for these answers.

REFERENCES

Campbell, D. and Stanley, J. (1966). *Experimental and quasi-experimental designs for research.* Chicago, Rand McNally.

Cook, T. D. and Campbell, D. T. (1979). *Quasi-experimental design and analysis issues for field settings.* Chicago, Rand McNally.

O'Sullivan, A. L. and Jacobsen, B. S. (1992). A randomized trial of a health care program for first-time adolescent mothers and their infants. *Nursing Research,* 41, 210-215.

10

Nonexperimental Designs

INTRODUCTION

Nonexperimental design can provide extensive amounts of data that can help fill in the gaps still found in nursing research. These designs help us clarify, see the real world, and assess relationships between variables, and they can provide clues to direct future, more controlled research. In this way, experimental and nonexperimental designs complement each other. Each provides necessary components of our lives. Nonexperimental designs allow us to discover some of the territory of nursing knowledge before trying to rearrange parts of it. It can be the base on which knowledge is built and further refined with experimental research.

LEARNING OBJECTIVES

On completion of this chapter, the student should be able to do the following:

- State the type of nonexperimental design used in a given study when provided the relevant sentences from the abstract or the report of research.
- Provide feasible explanations of the advantages and disadvantages of using nonexperimental design for a given situation.
- Specify the most appropriate type of nonexperimental design given specific research situations.
- Critique the use of nonexperimental design for specific studies.

ACTIVITY 1

Write a brief working definition of each of the following types of nonexperimental research designs. (Remember, a working definition needs to be in your own words.)

1. Correlational _____

   _____

2. Cross-sectional _____

   _____

3. Ex post facto _____

_____

4. Longitudinal _____

_____

5. Prediction _____

_____

6. Prospective _____

_____

7. Retrospective _____

_____

8. Survey _____

_____

Match the type of nonexperimental design in Column B with the appropriate phrase in Column A. Some terms from Column B will be used more than once.

Column A	Column B
9. _____ better known for breadth of data collected than depth	a. correlational
10. _____ a major disadvantage is the length of time needed for data collection	b. ex post facto c. cross-sectional
11. _____ main question is whether or not variable covary	d. longitudinal e. survey
12. _____ means "from after the fact"
13. _____ eliminate the confounding variable of maturation
14. _____ quantifies the magnitude and direction of a relationship
15. _____ collects data from the same group at several different points in time
16. _____ can be surprisingly accurate if sample is representative
17. _____ uses data from one point in time
18. _____ based on two or more naturally occurring groups with different conditions of the presumed independent variable

Check your answers with those in Appendix A, Chapter 10.

ACTIVITY 2

Your next task is to try to think like the researcher. Return to Chapter 10 in the text. Find the discussion pertaining to each of the nonexperimental designs listed at the beginning of Activity 1. Make a list of the advantages and disadvantages of each design.

1. Correlational:

   Advantages _____

   _____

   Disadvantages _____

   _____

2. Cross-sectional:

   Advantages _____

   _____

   Disadvantages _____

   _____

3. Ex post facto:

   Advantages _____

   _____

   Disadvantages _____

   _____

4. Longitudinal:

   Advantages _____

   _____

   Disadvantages _____

   _____

5. Prediction:

   Advantages _____

_____

Disadvantages _____

_____

6. Prospective:

Advantages _____

_____

Disadvantages _____

_____

7. Retrospective:

Advantages _____

_____

Disadvantages _____

_____

8. Survey

Advantages _____

_____

Disadvantages _____

_____

Check your answers with those in Appendix A, Chapter 10.

ACTIVITY 3

Each of the following studies gives indicators for the type of study being conducted and the purpose of the study. Remember, some studies use more than one type of nonexperimental design. For each of them list the type of design chosen, the advantages, and the disadvantages.

1. In this descriptive examination of student nurses' knowledge, attitudes, fears and phobias about persons with AIDS, 39 freshmen nursing students and 105 senior nursing students voluntarily participated in a study to ascertain if the educative program was moving them

toward the more humane treatment and care of these patients. The purpose of the study was to assess undergraduate nursing student's knowledge levels of the disease and their attitudes toward those who have been diagnosed with the disease. (Bryne and Murphy, 1993)

Type of design used _____

Pertinent advantages _____

_____

Pertinent disadvantages _____

_____

2. A descriptive study of women receiving hospital postpartum care was undertaken to determine whether or not these women exhibited the behaviors of taking-in and taking-hold defined by Reva Rubin and whether or not these behaviors and attitudes changed over time. The purpose was to ascertain if the subjects demonstrated taking-in and taking-hold behavior and attitudes based on a questionnaire and if these changed over the time of their hospitalization. (Ament, 1989)

Type of design used _____

Pertinent advantages _____

_____

Pertinent disadvantages _____

_____

3. The purpose of this exploratory, descriptive study was to describe the incarcerated pregnant woman and document her risk factors and pregnancy outcomes. Different instruments were used to assess risk factors, depressive symptomatology, and anxiety during the 3rd trimester and relate these to pregnancy outcome data. (Fogel, 1993)

Type of design used _____

Pertinent advantages _____

_____

Pertinent disadvantages _____

_____

4. The purpose of this study was to document skin changes in the nipple during the first week of breastfeeding in 20 Caucasian women and to explore the relationship of such changes to pain. Subjects were visited every 48 hours. Nipples were assessed and photo-

graphed, and the subjects were asked about the amount of pain they experienced. (Ziemer and Pigeon, 1993)

Type of design used _____

Pertinent advantages _____

_____

Pertinent disadvantages _____

_____

5. The purpose of this study was to determine the number of rubella-susceptible women who were clients of a family-planning clinic. The study involved a survey of the charts of all new clients seen in the clinic over a three-month period. (Eisele, 1993)

Type of design used _____

Pertinent advantages _____

_____

Pertinent disadvantages _____

_____

Check your answers with those in Appendix A, Chapter 10.

ACTIVITY 4

Read the following paragraphs about unwanted sexual experiences.

Nurses should be aware that many children and women have had perceived stressful sexual experiences that are kept in secret and have not been easily disclosed to a health professional. Words connoting abuse and victimization may be too strong, stereotypic, and emotionally laden for client usage, thus creating additional stress in assessment and treatment. Disclosure is related to the relationship of the offender and type of experience. Nurses need to be sensitive to the difficulty and risk that some women feel regarding disclosure.

Nurses need to be cognizant that family, neighbors, and friends, generally the persons considered as valuable social support, are the people most often involved in stressful, unwanted sexual experiences. "Double bind" situations should be acknowledged in treatment and prevention programs of stressful experiences of children and adolescents.

Why have stressful unwanted sexual experiences, including sexual abuse, exploitation, harassment, and victimization, taken so long to surface as a social and/or health problem? What are the specific events that constitute stressful unwanted sexual experiences that occur in childhood, adolescence, and adulthood? What have so many people who have had these experiences kept them secret from their closest confidants? What are the outcomes of these events? What are the relationships between victim and offender? These are complex questions, and much of the information about this phenomenon is speculative based on impressions or rather small clinical populations. (Mim and Chang, 1984)

Assume you are designing a study to address this situation. You want to consider several nonexperimental designs before deciding which design to use, so think through each of the designs listed. Now write brief descriptions of studies directed toward unwanted sexual experiences that will meet the criteria for each of the following types of nonexperimental design. "Brief" means no more than five sentences for each study. Only write the descriptions; do not worry about how realistic the resulting study would be. Refer to the text if you need to review the characteristics of any of the designs.

1. Survey _____

   _____

   _____

2. Correlational _____

   _____

   _____

3. Ex post facto _____

   _____

   _____

4. Prediction _____

   _____

   _____

5. Cross-sectional _____

   _____

   _____

6. Longitudinal _____

   _____

   _____

7. Retrospective _____

_____

_____

8. Prospective _____

_____

_____

Reread the described studies of unwanted sexual experience and answer the following questions:

1. Are any of the studies ethically unsound? Why?

_____

_____

2. How expensive in terms of time, actual dollars, and effort would you estimate each study to be? Rank them from the most expensive to the least.

_____

_____

3. How likely will subjects be to participate in each study? Would you?

_____

_____

_____

4. Which study would you like to see done?

_____

_____

_____

Check your answers with those in Appendix A, Chapter 10.

ACTIVITY 5

Your final task for this chapter is to critique the Grey, Cameron, and Thurber study (Appendix B in the text). Read the study and answer each of the 10 critique questions from Chapter 10 of the text.

1. Which nonexperimental design is utilized in the study?

   _____

2. Based on the theoretical framework, is the rational for the type of design evident? Explain.

   _____

3. Is the utilized design congruent with the purpose of the study?   Yes No

4. Is the utilized design appropriate for the research problem?   Yes No

5. Is the utilized design suited to the data collection methods?   Yes No

6. Does the researcher present the findings in a manner that is congruent with the utilized design?   Yes No

7. Does the researcher go beyond the relational parameters of the findings and erroneously infer cause-and-effect relationships between the variables? Explain.

   _____

8. Are there any reasons to believe that there are alternative explanations for the findings?

   _____

9. Where appropriate, how does the researcher discuss the threats to internal and external validity?

   _____

10. How does the author deal with the limitations of the study?

    _____

Check your answers with those in Appendix A, Chapter 10.

POSTTEST

1. _____ is the broadest category of nonexperimental design.

2. It can be further classified as _____ and

   _____.

3. The second major category of nonexperimental design according to LoBiondo-Wood and

   Haber is _____

4. The researcher is using _____ design when examining the
   relationship between two or more variables.

5. _____ designs have many similarities to quasi-experimental designs.

6. _____ design used in epideminological work is similar to
   ex post facto.

7. LoBiondo-Wood and Haber discuss four types of developmental studies. They are

   a) _____; b) _____;

   c) _____; and d) _____.

8. _____ studies data at one point in time while

   _____ collects data from the same group at different
   points in time.

9. A _____ study looks at presumed causes and moves
   forward in time to presumed effects.

10. The researcher is using a _____ design if she/he is trying to
    link present events to events that have occurred in the past.

The answers to the posttest are in the Instructor's Resource Manual. Please check with your
instructor for these answers.

REFERENCES

Ament, L. A. (1989). Maternal tasks of the puerperium reidentified. *JOGNN Nursing*, 19:330-
   335.
Byrne, V. A. and Murphy, J. F. (1993). Are we preparing future nurses to care for individuals
   with AIDS? *Journal of Nursing Education*, 32:84-86.
Eisele, C. J. (1993). Rubella susceptibility in women of childbearing age. *JOGNN Nursing*,
   22:260-263.

Fogel, C. I. (1992). Pregnant inmates: Risk factors and pregnancy outcomes. *JOGNN Nursing*, 22:33-39.

Ziemer, M. M. and Pigeon, J. G. (1993). Skin changes and pain the in the nipple during the 1st week of lactation. *JOGNN Nursing*, 22:247-256.

CHAPTER

11

Qualitative Approaches to Research

INTRODUCTION

Qualitative approaches to research are rapidly gaining in popularity as more holistic and comprehensive approaches to studying human phenomena than the more traditional quantitative research. Nurse researchers are discovering that qualitative research lends itself to studying the complexities of human beings and the response of humans to various life experiences. Being able to identify and interpret qualitative approaches to research and being able to differentiate it from quantitative research provides nurses with the opportunity to apply qualitative research reports to the practice of nursing.

LEARNING OBJECTIVES

On completion of this chapter, the student should be able to do the following:

- Distinguish the characteristics of qualitative research from those of quantitative research.
- Recognize the uses of qualitative research for nursing.
- Identify and differentiate the processes of phenomenological, ground theory, ethnographic, and historical critical methods.
- Use critiquing criteria to evaluate the qualitative research report.

ACTIVITY 1

Qualitative and quantitative research have distinct characteristics and differences. Once you are able to recognize the characteristics of qualitative research and differentiate it from quantitative research, you will be better able to interpret research report findings.

1. Complete the following statements related to qualitative research characteristics.

    a. Qualitative research is aimed at studying humans' experiences and realities through

    contact with individuals in their _____.

    b. Qualitative research embraces the notion that humans apply meaning to their life

    experiences and experiences evolve from _____.

c. The matrix of human-human-environment relationships which emerges daily is known

   as one's _____.

d. Qualitative researchers study individuals as they carry on their daily life activities in

   their _____ such as home, work, and school.

e. According to qualitative research approaches, humans are in a

   _____ with their environment.

f. Humans are thought to be unique individuals who dynamically interact with their

   environment and acquire personal experiences which are _____.

2. For the following research characteristics, put an **A** next to those indicative of a qualitative approach and a **B** next to those indicative of a quantitative approach.

   a. _____ Usually isolated in time
   b. _____ Studies humans in naturalistic settings
   c. _____ Measures one or more variables in a context-free setting
   d. _____ Truth is a subjective expression of reality
   e. _____ Truth is an objective expression of reality
   f. _____ Uses deductive analysis
   g. _____ Uses inductive analysis
   h. _____ Tests hypothesis
   i. _____ Generates hypothesis
   j. _____ Limits data collection by saturation
   k. _____ Determines sample size a-priori
   l. _____ Creates a description of human experiences

3. List the major elements in the quantitative approach to research on the left side of the page and list the major elements of the qualitative approach to research on the right side of the page. Discuss the similarities and differences of the two approaches with fellow students.

_____

_____

_____

_____

_____

_____

4. Describe which approach to research interests you more. Why?

_____

_____

_____

_____

_____

_____

_____

Check your answers with those in Appendix A, Chapter 11.

ACTIVITY 2

Qualitative research is conducive to nursing practice since its theoretical underpinnings closely approximate the philosophy of nursing.

1. Read the discussion and recommendation sections of the research report "Types and Meanings of Caring Behaviors Among Elderly Nursing Home Residents" by Hutchison and Bahr (1992) found in Appendix C of the text, and respond to the following items:

a. True   False   Caring is an important component in maintaining personal identity among nursing home residents.

b. True   False   For nursing home residents, being able to care for other humans affects their quality of life.

c. True   False   Hutchison's and Bahr's study was unable to validate previous studies on caring.

d. True   False   The study found that the ability and interest to care for other humans decrease as one ages.

e. True   False   The study supported Maslow's human needs theory relevant to a need for safety.

f. True   False   The study found that caring toward others helps nursing home residents to focus less on their own problems.

2. Qualitative research has many uses for nursing. After reading Hutchison's and Bahr's research report, list some other settings where this research could be carried out. Describe where you might like to replicate the study.

_____

_____

_____

_____

_____

_____

_____

_____

_____

_____

3. Leininger (1981) states that caring is the essence of nursing and Diers (1986) states "above all, nursing is caring" (p. 27). Describe how Hutchison's and Bahr's report supports these statements. Describe in what ways you use caring as part of your nursing practice.

_____

_____

_____

_____

_____

_____

_____

_____

_____

Check your answers with those in Appendix A, Chapter 11.

ACTIVITY 3

Four qualitative methods of research are the phenomenological, grounded theory, ethnographic, and historical methods.

1. For each characteristic listed below, indicate which method of qualitative research it
   describes. Use the abbreviations from the key provided.
   KEY: A = phenomenological   C = ethnographic
           B = grounded theory   D = historical

   a. _____ Uses primary and secondary sources
   b. _____ Uses "emic" and "etic" views of subjects' worlds
   c. _____ Research questions are action or change oriented
   d. _____ Central meanings arise from subjects' descriptions of lived experience
   e. _____ Truth is a lived experience
   f. _____ Uses theoretical sampling to analyze data
   g. _____ Discovers "domains" to analyze data
   h. _____ Provides insight on the past and serves as a guide to the present and future
   i. _____ Establishes fact, probability, or possibility
   j. _____ States individuals' history is a dimension of the present
   k. _____ Attempts to discover underlying social forces that shape human behavior
   l. _____ Interviews "key" informants
   m. _____ Presents data as a synthesized chronicle
   n. _____ Focuses on describing cultural groups
   o. _____ Establishes reliability through external and internal criticism
   p. _____ Researcher brackets his/her perspective
   q. _____ Subjects are currently experiencing a circumstance
   r. _____ Collects remembered information from subjects
   s. _____ Involves "field work"
   t. _____ Describes events from the past
   u. _____ May use photographs to describe current behavioral practices
   v. _____ Uses symbolic interaction as a theoretical base
   w. _____ Uses an inductive approach to understanding basic social processes

2. Read the research report "Types and Meanings of Caring Behaviors Among Elderly
   Nursing Home Residents" by Hutchison and Bahr (1991) found in Appendix C of the
   text, and complete the following multiple choice items:

   a. The qualitative method used in the research report is:

      (1) phenomenological
      (2) historical
      (3) ethnographic
      (4) grounded theory

   b. The social process being studied in the research report is:

      (1) the impact of senility
      (2) caring behaviors
      (3) activities of daily living
      (4) living in a nursing home

c. Data were gathered by way of:

    (1) observation and diaries
    (2) observation and measurement tools
    (3) observation and interviews
    (4) observation only

d. Which method was used to analyze data?

    (1) constant comparative analysis
    (2) taking photographs of subjects
    (3) Pearson r
    (4) asking subjects to recall their lived experience

e. Sample size was determined by:

    (1) a convenience sample of 20 subjects
    (2) the saturation method of 20 subjects
    (3) random selection from 117-bed facility
    (4) sample size is unimportant in this type of study

3. Of the four methods of qualitative research described in the text:

a. Select one method you find most interesting. _____

b. Explain why you find it interesting. _____

    _____

    _____

c. List 3-4 areas of study you might like to study using your selected method.

    _____

    _____

For example, you might want to study teenage mothers and you would like to use the grounded theory approach. You might like to know what it is like for teenagers to be mothers. Your research question might read:

How do teenage mothers manage their adolescent years, motherhood, and school and social lives?

d. Explain how you would collect data using the selected approach.

    _____

    _____

e. Describe how you would analyze the data (where appropriate to do so) or prepare the
final manuscript (if using the historical approach).

_____

_____

_____

f. Describe how the approach you selected could become part of your practice of nursing.

_____

_____

_____

Check your answers with those in Appendix A, Chapter 11.

ACTIVITY 4

Critiquing qualitative research enables the critiquer to make sense out of the research report
and build on a body of knowledge about human phenomena. Learning and applying the criteria for critiquing qualitative research is the first step in this process.

1. After reviewing the critiquing criteria from Chapter 11 in the text, complete the following.
   Match the step of the qualitative research process in Column B with the activity in
   Column A. Some steps from Column B will be used more than once.

	Column A	Column B
1. _____	the researcher's interpretation captured the participants' meaning	a. identifying phenomena
2. _____	participant consent was obtained	b. structuring the study
3. _____	there is a subject-phenomena relationship	c. researcher perspective
4. _____	data was synthesized	d. sample selection
5. _____	researcher bias is discussed	e. data gathering
6. _____	the qualitative method fits the research question	f. data analysis
7. _____	the phenomenon-human experience-natural setting relationship is established	g. describing findings
8. _____	the researcher described the participants' meaning of the phenomenon being studied	
9. _____	the context of the study is described in the research question	
10. _____	the analysis of the data is logically identified	

2. Using the 16 critiquing criteria from Chapter 11 in the text, evaluate Hutchison's and Bahr's report found in Appendix C of the text. Note which criteria are met and which criteria are not met. For each criterion, provide rationale for your answers.

Example:

Criterion 1. "Is the phenomenon focused on human experience within a natural setting?"

Yes. The phenomenon of caring behaviors is focused on nursing home residents. The authors explored and described the types and meanings of caring behaviors engaged in by elderly nursing home residents.

Criterion 2. "Is the phenomenon relevant to nursing and/or health?"

Yes. Caring is an integral part of the philosophy of nursing. Caring behaviors are considered vitally important in human growth and development, relationships, self-fulfillment, and health. It is a universal phenomenon which spans all cultures.

This is your opportunity to look critically at a research report and determine whether the criteria have been met.

_____

_____

_____

_____

_____

_____

_____

_____

_____

_____

_____

_____

_____

_____

_____

_____

_____

_____

_____

_____

_____

_____

3. After critiquing Hutchison's and Bahr's report, rate it for its overall performance. Assuming each criterion (1-16) in the critiquing criteria is weighted 6 points, grade the research report. The highest possible grade is 96.

_____

4. Select another qualitative research report from the literature and critique the report using the critiquing criteria from Chapter 11 in the text. Evaluate the report as you did with Hutchison's and Bahr's report.

_____

_____

_____

_____

_____

_____

_____

_____

_____

_____

_____

_____

_____

_____

_____

_____

_____

_____

_____

_____

_____

_____

_____

_____

_____

_____

_____

_____

5. Compare and contrast Hutchison's and Bahr's report with the report you selected to critique and answer the following questions:

   a. What are the similarities between the reports? (e.g., they both use the grounded theory method)

_____

_____

b. What are the differences?

_____

_____

c. Which report better meets the critiquing criteria?

_____

_____

d. Which report has more applicability to the practice of nursing? Why?

_____

_____

_____

e. Which report findings can you use in your particular practice of nursing?

_____

_____

_____

f. How would you use the preferred report's findings in your practice of nursing?

_____

_____

_____

Check your answers with those in Appendix A, Chapter 11.

POSTTEST

1. True   False   Qualitative research focuses on human experience in naturalistic settings.

2. True   False   Qualitative research is context-free.

3. The term *saturation* in qualitative research refers to:

    a. data repetition
    b. sample size
    c. research exhaustion
    d. subjects' exhaustion

4. In qualitative research, one way data are generally collected is by:

   a. questionnaires sent out to subjects
   b. surveys
   c. observation of subjects in natural settings
   d. interviewing subjects in a research laboratory

5. True   False   An example of a qualitative research question is: "Is maternal age related to the incidence of post partum depression?"

6. The qualitative research method which attempts to construct the meaning of human experience through persons who are living the experience is known as:

   a. phenomenologic
   b. historical
   c. grounded theory
   d. ethnographic

7. Qualitative researchers who seek to describe cultural groups would use which method of research?

   a. historical
   b. grounded theory
   c. phenomenologic
   d. ethnographic

8. Symbolic interaction is the theoretical base for which qualitative research method?

   a. phenomenologic
   b. grounded theory
   c. ethnographic
   d. historical

9. Describing the characteristics of American nurse leaders who lived between 1850 and 1900 is an example of which qualitative method?

   a. phenomenologic
   b. grounded theory
   c. historical
   d. ethnographic

10. True   False   External criticism in historical research relates to the authenticity of data sources.

The answers to the posttest are in the Instructor's Resource Manual. Please check with your instructor for these answers.

REFERENCES

Diers, D. (1986). To profess—To be a professional. *Journal of Nursing Administration*, 16, 25-30.

Hutchison, C. P. and Bahr, R. T. (1991). Types and meanings of caring behaviors among elderly nursing home residents. *Image: Journal of Nursing Scholarship*, 23(2), 85-88.

Leininger, M. (1984). *Care: An essential human need. Proceedings of three national caring conferences* (pp. 5-20). Thorofare, NJ: Charles B. Slack.

Leininger, M. (1984). *Care: The essence of nursing and health*. Thorofare, NJ: Charles B. Slack.

12

Sampling

INTRODUCTION

Sampling consists of choosing those elements to be used in answering the research question. The ideal sampling strategy is one in which the elements truly represent the population while controlling for any source of bias. Reality modulates the ideal. Considerations of efficiency, practicality, ethics, and availability frequently alter the ideal sampling strategy for a given study.

LEARNING OBJECTIVES

On completion of this chapter, the student should be able to do the following:

- List the advantages and disadvantages of the following sampling strategies:
  a. convenience sampling
  b. quota sampling
  c. purposive sampling
  d. simple random sampling
  e. stratified random sampling
  f. cluster sampling
  g. systematic sampling
- Distinguish between probability and nonprobability sampling strategies.
- Identify the sampling strategy used in example studies.
- Evaluate the congruence between the sample used and population of interest.
- Critique the sampling component of a study.

ACTIVITY 1

For each of the sampling strategies introduced in Chapter 12 of the text, list the major advantage and the major disadvantage in its use.

1. Convenience sampling:

   Advantage _____

   Disadvantage _____

2. Quota sampling:

   Advantage _____

   Disadvantage _____

3. Purposive sampling:

   Advantage _____

   Disadvantage _____

4. Simple random sampling:

   Advantage _____

   Disadvantage _____

5. Stratified random sampling:

   Advantage _____

   Disadvantage _____

6. Cluster sampling:

   Advantage _____

   Disadvantage _____

7. Systematic sampling:

   Advantage _____

   Disadvantage _____

Check your answers with those in Appendix A, Chapter 12.

ACTIVITY 2

Identify the category of sampling for each of the following sampling strategies. Use the abbreviations from the key provided.

KEY: P = Probability sampling
       N = Nonprobability sampling

1. _____ Simple random sampling
2. _____ Purposive sampling
3. _____ Cluster sampling
4. _____ Quota sampling

5. _____ Convenience sampling
6. _____ Systematic sampling
7. _____ Stratified random sampling

Check your answers with those in Appendix A, Chapter 12.

ACTIVITY 3

For each of the following examples of studies, identify the sampling strategy used.

1. The sample for the study of critical thinking behavior of undergraduate baccalaureate nursing students consisted of students enrolled in junior and senior level courses in three schools of nursing. In each program, students were invited to participate until a total sample representing 10% of the junior level students and 10% of the senior level students was obtained.

   _____

2. Every eighth person on the diabetic clinic patient roster was asked to participate in the study. A table of random numbers was used to select the beginning of the sampling within the first sampling interval.

   _____

3. Using a table of random numbers, the sample consisting of 50 clients was selected from the list of all postpartum mothers receiving public health nursing care during the first six months of 1993.

   _____

4. The sample consisted of all patients ages 30 to 60 enrolled in a cardiac rehabilitation program.

   _____

5. To select the sample, 25 rehabilitation centers were randomly selected from the list of all rehabilitation centers in the United States. Ten nurses were randomly selected from each site for a final sample of 250 nurses.

   _____

6. The study of arthritis self-care was conducted with clients attending an arthritis support group.

   _____

7. In order to study educational opportunities for nurses from various ethnic groups, a list of all nurses in the state of California was sorted by ethnicity. The sample consisted of 10%

of the nurses in each ethnic group, selected according to a table of random numbers.

Check your answers with those in Appendix A, Chapter 12.

ACTIVITY 4

Using the critiquing criteria listed in Chapter 12, critique the sample selected for the study by Stewart Fahs and Kinney located in the appendix of the text.

1. _____

2. _____

3. _____

4 _____

5. _____

6. _____

7. _____

8. _____

9. _____

10 _____

11. _____

12. _____

Check your answers with those in Appendix A, Chapter 12.

POSTTEST

Read the description of this sample and answer the questions which follow.

A random sample of 50 families was selected from the pediatric clinic roster of 450 families. The demographic data of the families were compared to the demographic data of the entire clinic roster in terms of language, ethnicity, age and number of children, and primary diagnoses for most recent clinic visits. Using t-tests and Chi Square, there were no statistically significant differences in demographic variables. Each of the families received a survey and participated in an interview regarding satisfaction with care received from the nurse practitioner. The final sample consisted of 45 families; 5 families had moved and had no forwarding address. The sample families had 1 to 5 children, with a mean of 2. Ages of children ranged from infants to 18 years, with a mean age of 6 years. All families spoke English as first or second language. Ethnicity was 80% white, 10% Hispanic, and 10% other.

1. Has the sample been adequately described?

   _____

2. How do the sample characteristics correspond to the larger population?

   _____

3. How was the sample selected? Is this a probability or nonprobability sample?

   _____

4. Is this sample size appropriate?

   _____

The answers to the posttest are in the Instructor's Resource Manual. Please check with your instructor for these answers.

REFERENCE

Stewart Fahs, P. S. and Kinney, M. R. (1991). The abdomen, thigh, and arm as sites for subcutaneous sodium heparin injections. *Nursing Research*, 40(4): 204-207.

13

Legal-Ethical Issues

INTRODUCTION

Patient advocacy is one of the primary roles of a professional nurse. Nowhere is this more necessary than in the field of research. The nurse must be the client advocate, whether acting as the researcher, a participant in research, or a provider of care for research subjects. Legal and ethical issues abound in research, and the nurse must be not only aware of them but capable of assessing and evaluating them. Nurses must be cognizant of Institutional Review Boards, their role, and the federal regulations on which they base their decisions.

LEARNING OBJECTIVES

On completion of this chapter, the student should be able to do the following:

- Appraise, within given clinical situations, the adequacy of the informed consent process.
- Identify the existence or absence of critical nursing behaviors when enacting the role of the client advocate given a clinical research situation.
- Practice decision making skills as a member of an Institutional Review Board.
- Evaluate the legal and ethical responsibilities of the professional nurse as a researcher in a given clinical situation.

ACTIVITY 1

Examine the following three excerpts from informed consent forms and decide if they adequately meet the criteria necessary for informed consent as described in "Guidelines for Informed Consent" in Chapter 13 of the text.

1. "If you have any questions about this research or about any consequences that occur as a result of your participation in the research, please contact the researcher at the university."

   Is this an adequate explanation? Would you sign the consent form with this clause in it? If not, what would make it adequate to meet the criteria described in the guidelines?

   _____

   _____

2. "There may be risks to the use of this new treatment; however, we do not want to tell you about them in advance. We are concerned that if we tell you what we anticipate the side effects might be, you will develop them through the self-fulfillment prophecy. If something unusual should happen once you have started this new protocol, please notify us."

Is this an adequate explanation? Would you sign the consent form with this clause in it? If not, what would make it adequate to meet the criteria described in the guidelines?

_____

_____

3. "Your anonymity and confidentiality will be protected when the results of this research are reported. Once you enter the study, you will be given an identifying number, and this will be used in all data analysis. The original consent forms with accompanying assigned numbers will be kept in a locked cabinet in the Department of Nursing Research Office and will be destroyed on completion of the study. Furthermore, data will be reported only as group data."

Is this an adequate explanation? Would you sign the consent form with this clause in it? If not, what would make it adequate to meet the criteria described in the guidelines?

_____

_____

Read the following situations involving informed consent forms and answer the questions regarding each.

4. As you are making your rounds at the beginning of the shift, you notice one of your primary care patients, who has a diagnosis of hemophilia, arguing loudly with his wife over a piece of paper. He's claiming, "If I participate in this study, I will be given preferential treatment, and I'll get this experimental drug that I wouldn't get a chance to get otherwise." The wife responds, "I don't think that is what this means. I think some people will get the experimental drug and others will not, and you won't even know which group you are in." He responds, "No, no, no—you've got it all wrong again. The doc said I'd be part of an experiment; that means for sure I'll get to try the new drug." The wife looks up at you and says, "Nurse, can you help us understand this form?" She hands you the following:

Human Subjects Participation Consent Form

The purpose of this study is to test a new drug for the treatment of AIDS in contrast with the traditional methods of treatment. The drug has been tested extensively with animals with positive results; however, this will be the first test series with humans. If you agree to participate in the research you will be randomly assigned to one of two groups, the experimental group (receiving the new drug — Anging) or the control group receiving the traditional treatment. Each group will receive one injection per day, but even your nurse will not be told which group you are in or which of the medications (traditional or experimental) you will be receiving.

The possible risks to you, if you choose to participate, include side effects from the new drug as yet unknown but which could include allergic reactions, skin rash, hair loss, and gastrointestinal ulcers, as well as even more severe reactions. If you choose to participate and are assigned to the control group, one risk is that you might become depressed once the study is over and it is revealed that you have been in the control group.

The possible benefits are that the experimental drug may prove more effective in controlling your illness than traditional therapy. If you choose not to participate in this study, however, your treatment at this hospital will not be jeopardized; you will continue to receive the same treatment you have been receiving.

If you have any questions about this study, please contact the researcher at any time at the address listed below. You will be given a copy of this consent form with the researcher's address and phone number on it. You are free to withdraw your participation at any time without prejudice to yourself. There will be no payment given for your participation in the study, nor will there be any additional expenses if you participate in the study. Extra studies will be done on the blood routinely drawn from you, but the research project will pay for these tests.

All information given by you will be kept confidential, and your identity will not be revealed at any time.

On the basis of the above statements, I agree to participate in the research project.

_____   _____
Participant's signature   Investigator's signature

_____   1234 Old Chemistry Hall
Date   Newton Medical Center
                                                                 Newton, CA 94023
                                                                 (415) 123-4567

Explain how you as a nurse patient advocate would intervene in this situation:

_____

_____

_____

5. On your unit, clinical research trials are taking place testing a new procedure for injecting a drug that is extremely irritating to tissues. In the control group, this drug is being administered by the Z technique to minimize tissue damage and discomfort. In the experimental group, the drug is being administered by the X technique. It is the third day of the testing. The clients who are in the experimental group are complaining of extreme pain after each injection. You examine the injection sites and notice redness, heat, and

oozing clear fluid from the area. Several patients in the experimental group ask you if any-thing can be done to stop these really painful injections. In your role as client advocate, what nursing interventions will you make? What is your rationale for your actions?

_____

_____

_____

6. You are working in a drug and alcohol treatment center in southern California where many well-known people are admitted for treatment. A new detoxification regime, con-sisting primarily of diet and exercise rather than gradual withdrawal of the abused sub-stance, is being tested, and many of the patients have been asked to sign consent forms to participate in this program. The consent form states that the patient's name may be used when the results of this research are reported in medical journals. When a patient asks you if he must participate and why they have to use his name, how will you respond?

_____

_____

_____

Check your answers with those in Appendix A, Chapter 13.

ACTIVITY 2

In the following situations, put yourself in the position of being the staff nurse member of a seven-member hospital institutional review board. Your task is to review proposals from re-searchers asking to conduct research within your hospital. Rate each of the three proposals as being minimum, moderate, or maximum risk to the patients and then decide whether you would give permission for the research to be conducted in your institution. The Code of Fed-eral Regulations outlines the criteria to be used when evaluating research proposals. You need to read each situation, think about each of the eight criteria, and decide whether or not the researchers correctly balanced the risk of the research with the safeguards provided.

Code of Federal Regulations

1. Risks to subjects are minimized.
2. Risks to subjects are reasonable in relation to anticipated benefits.
3. Selection of the subjects is equitable.
4. Informed consent (in one of several possible forms) must be sought from each pro-spective subject or the subject's legally authorized representative.
5. Informed consent must be properly documented.
6. Where appropriate, the research plan makes adequate provision for monitoring the data collected to ensure subjects' safety.
7. Where appropriate, there are adequate provisions to protect the privacy of subjects and the confidentiality of data.

8. Where some or all of the subjects are likely to be vulnerable to coercion or undue influence, such as persons who are economically or educationally disadvantaged, appropriate additional safeguards are included.

1. Study A is designed to observe the level-of-orientation response of hospitalized geriatric patients to the presence of pets. The researchers proposed to take several units in a nursing home and request all ambulatory patients who are oriented enough to be able to read and understand a consent form to participate in the study. Each patient will be given a copy of the consent form, which includes a phone number in case they wish to withdraw from the study at any time. Those who agree to participate will be randomly divided into control and experimental groups. Before any interventions all subjects will have their level of orientation tested twice a day for two weeks.

   a. Based on the eight criteria, list the number of each criteria (1-8) adequately met in this study.

   _____

   b. List those numbers (1-8) that this study does not safeguard or that are not mentioned.

   _____

   c. Would you rate this proposal as being of minimum, moderate, or maximum risk to

   patients? _____

   d. Will you allow this study to be conducted at this institution?   Yes   No

2. Study B. In the outpatient OB clinics of your hospital several staff members have noted that an increasing number of patients are in the 15- to 18-year-old age group. Adolescents come to this clinic because it is the only free clinic available in their area, and they state they cannot afford to see a private doctor. This clinic is their only option for health care. The nurses in the clinic designed a study that will gather data from the adolescents themselves and their peers at the high school. The study is an attempt to determine what socio-cultural changes might be causing this sudden increase in adolescent pregnancies.

   The nurses do not intend to use a written consent form because they think the prospective mothers and their peers would be reluctant to sign anything, and it would be difficult to write one in a language the adolescents could understand. Instead they will say to each student, "We are nurses from XYZ hospital and we would like to ask you a few questions." To find the pregnant adolescent's peers they will go to her high school and attempt to interview three or four other students in her grade.

   a. Based on the eight criteria, list the number of each criteria (1-8) adequately met in this study.

   _____

b. List those numbers (1-8) that this study does not safeguard or that are not mentioned.

_____

c. Would you rate this proposal as being of minimum, moderate, or maximum risk to

patients? _____

d. Will you allow this study to be conducted at this institution?   Yes   No

3. Study C is proposed by a group of graduate students in exercise physiology. As the experimental group they want to use patients from the cardiac unit and from the hospital's cardiac rehabilitation clinic to determine the patients' outer limits of exercise capability. They propose to use students from the university and test the outer limits of their exercise capability as a control group. Their rationale is that from personal observations while assisting on the cardiac rehabilitation units, they have noted that the focus is on the minimum amount of exercise to be performed without signs and symptoms of distress by these patients. They conclude from the questions they receive that the patients should be shown what their maximum limits are while in a safe place (the hospital) and then they will be able to exercise more freely when home. They will use a written consent form that will explain the benefits of the program to the prospective subjects.

a. Based on the eight criteria, list the number of each criteria (1-8) adequately met in this study.

_____

b. List those numbers (1-8) that this study does not safeguard or that are not mentioned.

_____

c. Would you rate this proposal as being of minimum, moderate, or maximum risk to

patients? _____

d. Will you allow this study to be conducted at this institution?   Yes   No

Check your answers with those in Appendix A, Chapter 13.

ACTIVITY 3

Identify the methods for complying with informed consent in the three articles provided in Appendices A, B, and C of the textbook.

1. Heparin injections _____

2. Diabetic children _____

3. Caring in elderly _____

Check your answers with those in Appendix A, Chapter 13.

ACTIVITY 4

List the three ethical principles relevant to conduct of research involving human subjects.

1. _____

2. _____

3. _____

Check your answers with those in Appendix A, Chapter 13.

ACTIVITY 5

Identify at least four categories of subjects who are vulnerable or have diminished autonomy.

1. _____

2. _____

3. _____

4. _____

Check your answers with those in Appendix A, Chapter 13.

POSTTEST

1. How can researchers maintain anonymity and confidentiality for the patients involved in a research project?

    _____

2. If a researcher does not give a name, address, and telephone number where he can be reached if a patient wishes to withdraw from a study or report complications, is this an adequate consent form that you would encourage a client to sign?   Yes   No

3. Should a researcher list all the possible risks and benefits of participating in a research study?   Yes   No

4. If you question whether a researcher has permission to conduct a study in your hospital, you would ask her to show you approval from what group?

    _____

5. If you agreed to collect data for a researcher who had not asked the patient's permission to participate in the research study, you would be violating the patient's right to:

_____

6. Where would the reader of research generally find information related to informed consent and the rights of human subjects?

_____

7. Briefly discuss the differences between *assent* and *consent*.

_____

_____

_____

_____

8. Are researchers who are operating under exempt status released from obtaining informed consent?   Yes   No

The answers to the posttest are in the Instructor's Resource Manual. Please check with your instructor for these answers.

REFERENCES

Costa, L. M. (1991). Competency and consent. *Geriatric Nursing*, 12, 254.

Flarey, D. L. (1992). Legal and ethical issues in HIV testing. *Journal of Nursing Administration*, 22, 14-20.

Reid, J. (1991). Informed consent: An ethical dilemma. *British Journal of Theatre of Nursing*, 2, 23-25.

Smith, A. M. (1993). Consent to treatment in childhood. *Archives of Disease in Childhood*, 67, 1247-1248.

Tarmmelleo, A. D. (1992). Patient sues nurse for failure to obtain informed consent. *Regan Report in Nursing Law*, 33, 4.

CHAPTER

14

Data Collection Methods

INTRODUCTION

This chapter focuses on basic information about data collection. The intent is to provide the reader with a basis to evaluate and critique data collection methods in published research studies. The methods used to collect data about the phenomenon of interest are varied. Readers should be prepared to ask questions about the appropriateness of the measures chosen by the researcher to gather data about the variable of concern.

LEARNING OBJECTIVES

On completion of this chapter, the student should be able to do the following:

- Describe the types of data collection methods used in nursing research.
- Identify whether a data collection measure is an example of:
  a. a physiological measure
  b. an observational measure
  c. an interview measure
  d. a questionnaire
  e. records or available data
- Analyze the strengths and limitations of specified data collection instruments.
- Critique data collection components of the methodology of given studies.
- Critically evaluate the utilization potential of published research studies based upon a critique of their data collection methods.

ACTIVITY 1

Read the following vignette:

A principal of a metropolitan high school is concerned about reports of an increasing number of male teenage drug-users within the school. Rumors have suggested that the school bathrooms play a central role in the students' ability to obtain and use drugs while they are in school. The principal has a nephew who is a university student and who recently asked for assistance in identifying an idea for a research project for a psychology class. The principal mentions that it would be helpful to have a study done of the traffic flow in and out of the men's bathroom (who goes in and how often), as well as some direct observations to determine the level of drug use in the bathroom. The university student is told that he could (a) conduct his study during spring break from the university; (b) attend the high school as a new transfer student; and (c) be assigned as a hall monitor to complete the research project. The nephew agrees.

You are working as the school nurse. When you see John, the nephew, standing at the end of the hall, you recognize that he is new in the school and ask him what he is doing. He goes to your office, explains his research project, and requests your cooperation (i.e., silence).

1. Which data collection method is used in the vignette?

   a. a physiological measure
   b. an observational measure
   c. an interview measure
   d. a questionnaire
   e. records or available data

2. Which of the four types of concealment is used in this study?

   a. concealment without intervention
   b. concealment with intervention
   c. no concealment without intervention
   d. no concealment with intervention

3. In your role as school nurse, how will you respond?

   a. You decide not to expose his study but ask for the results so that you can use the information about the specific drugs in use to develop antidrug lectures.
   b. You call the superintendent of schools and explain to him what is occurring.
   c. You tell John and the principal that they are conducting an unethical research project because they do not have the consent of the participants and the approval of the parents or an Institutional Review Board.

4. Briefly explain the rationale for your choice of intervention in the above question.

_____

_____

Check your answers with those in Appendix A, Chapter 14.

ACTIVITY 2

Review the three articles referenced below; be especially thorough in reading the sections that deal with data collection methods. Answer the questions in relation to what you discover in these three articles. For some questions, there may be more than one answer.

Grey, M., Cameron, M. E., and Thurber, F. W. (1991). Coping and adaptation in children with diabetes. *Nursing Research*, 40(3), 144-149. (Appendix B of the text)

1. Which data collection method is used in this research study?

    a. a physiological measure
    b. an observational measure
    c. an interview measure
    d. a questionnaire
    e. records or available data

Hutchison, C. P. and Bahr, R. T. (1991). Types and meanings of caring behaviors among elderly nursing home residents. *Image: Journal of Nursing Scholarship*, 23(2), 85-88. (Appendix C of the text)

2. Which data collection method is used in this research study?

    a. a physiological measure
    b. an observational measure
    c. an interview measure
    d. a questionnaire
    e. records or available data

3. Which of the four types of concealment is used in this study?

    a. concealment without intervention
    b. concealment with intervention
    c. no concealment without intervention
    d. no concealment with intervention

Stewart Fahs, P. S. and Kinney, M. R. (1991). The abdomen, thigh, and arm as sites for sub-cutaneous sodium heparin injections. *Nursing Research*, 40(4), 204-207. (Appendix A of the text)

4. Which data collection method is used in this research study?

    a. a physiological measure
    b. an observational measure
    c. an interview measure
    d. a questionnaire
    e. records or available data

Check your answers with those in Appendix A, Chapter 14.

ACTIVITY 3

Using the content of Chapter 14 in the text, circle the correct response for each question. Some questions will have more than one answer.

1. In nursing research, when might physiological measures of data collection be especially useful?

a. for identification of biobehavioral interface

b. when one wants to determine the effectiveness of particular nursing actions

c. if one is interested in the measurement of metabolic indicators

d. all of the above

2. Which of the following would be considered advantages of using physiological measures as data collection methods?

a. the ease in execution of the measures

b. the unlikeliness that study subjects can distort the physiological information

c. their objectivity, precision, and sensitivity

d. all of the above

3. Which of the following would be considered disadvantages of using physiological measures as data collection methods?

a. some instruments are inexpensive

b. use of the instrument may at times change the variable being measured

c. measuring devices may be altered by environmental factors

d. instruments may require specialized knowledge and training for their use

4. In nursing research, when might observational measures of data collection be especially useful?

a. when the number of subjects in a study is extremely large

b. if the researcher is interested in the ways the subjects react under specific circumstances

c. in complex research situations when it is difficult to separate the processes or interactions

d. when the researcher is interested in character traits or behaviors

5. Which of the following would be considered advantages of using observational data collection methods?

a. observational methods may consume many of the researchers' resources

b. observational methods are generally easy to implement and do not require specialized skills

c. observational methods may be the only way to study the variable of interest

d. observational methods could be used in either experimental or nonexperimental designs in laboratory studies

6. Which of the following would be considered disadvantages of using observational data collection methods?

a. individual bias may interfere with the data collection

b. ethical concerns may be increasingly significant to researchers using observational data collection methods

c. individual judgments and values influence the perceptions of the observers

d. all of the above

7. In nursing research, when might interviews be used as an appropriate method for data collection?

   a. when the researcher is interested in a personal account
   b. when the researcher wants to know about the subjects' personal beliefs
   c. when the researcher wants to gather unbiased information
   d. all of the above

8. Which of the following would be considered advantages of using interviews for data collection in nursing research?

   a. interviews provide the researcher with the opportunity to gather rich information
   b. interviews provide the opportunity to clarify questions
   c. interviews provide a means to gather information from some subjects (e.g., children, the blind, the illiterate) that might not be able to be obtained by other methods
   d. all of the above

9. Which of the following would be considered disadvantages of using interviews for data collection in nursing research?

   a. data gathered through interviews may reflect what the subject thinks the researcher wants to hear rather than what the subject believes to be true
   b. an interviewer may influence the subjects' responses by the manner in which the interview is conducted
   c. interviews provide data that reflects the individual participant's perceptions
   d. all of the above

10. In nursing research, when might questionnaires be used as an appropriate method for data collection?

    a. whenever expense is a concern for the researcher
    b. when a researcher is interested in obtaining information directly from the subjects
    c. when the researcher needs to collect data from a large group of subjects that are not easily accessible
    d. when accuracy is of the utmost importance to the researcher

11. Which of the following would be considered advantages of using questionnaires as a data collection method?

    a. when the researcher is interested in ascertaining information about the subjects' beliefs and attitudes
    b. when expense is a concern for the researcher
    c. whenever the researcher wants to assure individual subjects that their responses will remain anonymous
    d. all of the above

12. Which of the following would be considered disadvantages of using questionnaires as a data collection method?

    a. multiple measures can be used in a research study to study a variable of interest
    b. study participants may fail to carefully read the questions prior to marking their responses
    c. subjects may fail to interpret questions as the researcher intended
    d. research subjects may not do a thorough job in answering the questions or returning them to the researcher within the specified time frame

13. In nursing research, what type of nursing problems would be especially suited to the use of available records or data?

    a. when asking specific research questions for which data already exist
    b. when the researcher merely wants to summarize existing data
    c. when there are existing records or data that might be used to answer research questions in a new way
    d. all of the above

14. Which of the following would be considered advantages of using existing records or available data to answer a research question?

    a. the use of available data reduces the likelihood of researcher bias in data collection
    b. time involvement in the research study can be reduced by the use of available records or data
    c. consistent collection of information over periods of time allows the researcher to study trends
    d. all of the above

15. Which of the following would be considered disadvantages of using existing records or available data to answer a research question?

    a. the researcher does not have to identify individual participants for the study
    b. the researcher may be unable to identify if records have been collected or saved in a biased manner
    c. institutions may be reluctant to allow a researcher access to existing records or data
    d. accuracy and thoroughness in the collection of data may be difficult to determine

Check your answers with those in Appendix A, Chapter 14.

ACTIVITY 4

The *first task* in this activity is to consider the strengths and limitations of each strategy. Availability and accessibility concerns? Validity concerns and possibilities? The utility of the strategy (e.g., cost in time, money, special skills or training needed)? Value in addressing the purpose of the study? Use information presented in this and previous chapters to thoroughly consider and valuate each strategy.

The *second task* is to design an appropriate data collection methodology. You may use any one strategy or a combination of the strategies listed. You also may feel free to develop new ones. Explain the reasoning behind your choices in terms of practicality, validity, utility, protection of participants, and any special knowledge you may have. Before you begin this task, first identify the independent and dependent variables and restate the purpose of the study in the form of a question.

Example Research Situation to use for Exercises 1 and 2

The purpose of the study is to evaluate the effectiveness of an inservice program for nurses who work closely with post-myocardial infarction (post-MI) clients. The program was designed to help nurses develop new skills in facilitating the discussion of post-MI sexual activity.

Exercise 1

Read each of the suggested strategies, identify the type of data collection method which is implied, and then consider the strengths and weaknesses of the strategy.

1. Pre- and post-test given at the time of the inservice program, which questions the nurses' knowledge about relevant physiogical aspects of the client post-MI and sexual activity.

   a. Data collection method

   _____

   b. Strengths of strategy

   _____

   c. Limitations of strategy

   _____

2. Pre- and post-inservice program interview regarding the nurses' feelings about discussing sex with a post-MI client and/or relevant significant other.

   a. Data collection method

   _____

   b. Strengths of strategy

   _____

   c. Limitations of strategy

   _____

3. Survey of post-MI clients' knowledge and feelings regarding sexual activity on the day of discharge.

   a. Data collection method

   _____

   b. Strengths of strategy

   _____

   c. Limitations of strategy

   _____

4. Pre- and post-test inservice program videotape of each nurse discussing sexual activity with a post-MI client and/or relevant significant other.

   a. Data collection method

   _____

   b. Strengths of strategy

   _____

   c. Limitations of strategy

   _____

5. Pre- and post-test inservice program videotape of each nurse role-playing a discussion of sexual activity with a post-MI client and/or relevant significant other.

   a. Data collection method

   _____

   b. Strengths of strategy

   _____

   c. Limitations of strategy

   _____

6. Structured interview on the date of an eight-week post-MI stress ECG with the post-MI client and/or relevant significant other regarding resumption of sexual activity.

a. Data collection method

_____

b. Strengths of strategy

_____

c. Limitations of strategy

_____

7. Pre- and post-inservice program audiotape of each nurse discussing sexual activity with a post-MI client and/or relevant significant other.

a. Data collection method

_____

b. Strengths of strategy

_____

c. Limitations of strategy

_____

Exercise 2

Design an appropriate data collection methodology for the Example Research Situation. Use your critical thinking skills to evaluate the appropriateness in choosing one or more of the above strategies identified in Exercise 1. Feel free to create a new strategy or to combine several methods. Be prepared to support your choice.

1. What is the dependent variable?   _____

2. What is the independent variable?   _____

3. State the research question.

_____

4. What is the best method for data collection?

_____

5. What is your rationale for choice of data collection method?

_____

_____

Check your answers with those in Appendix A, Chapter 14.

ACTIVITY 5

Read the descriptive material for each of the following studies and identify the type of data collection method used. Although only a brief descriptor for each research study is provided, use your analytical skills to determine the strategy used for data collection. Support your answer with a brief rationale for why you think the researchers chose this particular method. If you would like to read the complete studies, refer to the reference section at the end of this chapter for the citation.

Case 1

Hahn, Ro, Song, Kim, Kim, and Yoo (1993) studied the effectiveness of using biofeedback training and progressive muscle relaxation therapy in patients with essential hypertension. A treatment group received both interventions, but the control group received only the muscle relaxation therapy. Blood pressures were measured prior to any treatment in both groups.

1. Data collection method used _____

2. Rationale for choice _____

_____

Case 2

There is an increasing concern about the potential for elder mistreatment by their caregivers. A study by Sayles-Cross (1993) considered the perceptions of the caregivers of elder adults. The researcher was especially interested in the consequences of the caring, the conflict and stress experienced by the caregiver, and the caregiving role itself.

1. Data collection method used _____

2. Rationale for choice _____

_____

Case 3

Nurses conducting qualitative research studies have been concerned that they are at a disadvantage when being considered for funding of their work. Cohen, Knafl, and Dzurec (1993) studied the evaluation of qualitative research grants. They conducted their study based upon a convenience sample of summary statements of reviews of 19 grant proposals.

1. Data collection method used _____

2. Rationale for choice _____

_____

Case 4

Generally, it is considered therapeutic for survivors of incest to have opportunities to tell their story. Nurses encounter these individuals within a variety of practice settings but may be insensitive to their lived experience. Kondora (1993) conducted a phenomenological study of adult women survivors of childhood incest.

1. Data collection method used _____

2. Rationale for choice _____

_____

Case 5

Ragsdale, Kotarba, and Morrow (1992) used a grounded theory methodology to study the quality of life in persons with AIDS during hospitalization. One method used to gather data for the study was semi-structured interviews which were audiotaped. The researchers also spent 62 hours in the unit.

1. Data collection method used _____

2. Rationale for choice _____

_____

Check your answers with those in Appendix A, Chapter 14.

POSTTEST

Read each question thoroughly and then circle the correct answer. For some questions more than one answer may be correct.

1. The process of translating concepts that are of interest to the researcher into observable and measurable phenomena is known as:

   a. objectivism
   b. systematization
   c. subjectivism
   d. operationalization

2. Answering research questions pertaining to psychosocial variables can best be answered by using which data gathering technique(s)?

   a. observation
   b. interviews
   c. questionnaires
   d. all of the above

3. Collection of data from each subject in the same or in a similar manner is known as:

   a. repetition
   b. dualism
   c. consistency
   d. recidivism

4. Consistency of observations between two or more observers is known as:

   a. intrarater reliability
   b. interrater reliability
   c. consistency reliability
   d. repetitive reliability

5. Physiological and biological measurement might be used by nurse researchers when studying which of these variables?

   a. a comparison of student nurses' ACT scores and their GPAs
   b. hypertensive clients' responses to a stress test
   c. children's dietary patterns
   d. the degree of pain relief achieved following guided imagery

6. Scientific observations should fulfill which of the following conditions?

   a. observations are consistent with the study objectives
   b. observations are standardized and systematically recorded
   c. observations are checked and controlled
   d. all of the above

7. In a research study, a participant observer spent regularly scheduled hours in a homeless shelter and occasionally stayed overnight. The persons staying in the home were told that this person was conducting a research study. The researcher freely engaged in conversation and openly observed the homeless. What is the observational role of the researcher?

   a. concealment without intervention
   b. concealment with intervention
   c. no concealment without intervention
   d. no concealment with intervention

8. In unstructured observation, which of the following might occur?

   a. extensive field notes are recorded
   b. subjects are informed what behaviors are being observed
   c. the researcher frequently records interesting anecdotes
   d. all of the above

9. Which of the following is not consistent with a Likert scale?

   a. it contains close-ended items
   b. it contains open-ended items
   c. it contains lists of statements
   d. items are evaluated on the amount of agreement

10. Although it is acceptable to use multiple instruments within a research study, the study is more acceptable if only one method is used for the data collection.

    a. True
    b. False

11. Social desirability is seldom a concern for researchers when the data collection method used in the study is interviews.

    a. True
    b. False

12. A researcher desires to use a questionnaire in a study but cannot find one that will gather the information desired about a particular variable. The decision is made to develop a new instrument. Which of the following should the researcher do?

    a. define the construct, formulate the items, and assess the items for content validity
    b. develop instructions for users and pilot the instrument
    c. estimate reliability and validity
    d. all of the above

13. The researcher who invests significant amounts of time in the development of an instrument has a professional responsibility to publish the results.

    a. True
    b. False

14. In order to evaluate the adequacy of various data collection methods, which of the following should be observed in the written research report?

    a. clear identification of the rationale for selecting a physiological measure
    b. the problems of bias and reactivity are addressed with observational measures
    c. there is a clear explanation of how interviews were conducted and how interviewers were trained
    d. all of the above

15. In conducting a research study, the researcher has a responsibility to ensure that all study subjects received the same information and data was collected from all participants in the same manner.

    a. True
    b. False

The answers to the posttest are in the Instructor's Resource Manual. Please check with your instructor for these answers.

REFERENCES

Cohen, M. Z., Knafl, K., and Dzurec, L. C. (1993). Grant writing for qualitative research. *Image: Journal of Nursing Scholarship*, 25(2), 151-156.

Hahn, Y. B., Ro, Y. J., Song, H. H., Kim, N. C., Kim, H. S., and Yoo, Y. S. (1993). The effect of thermal biofeedback and progressive muscle relaxation training in reducing blood pressure of patients with essential hypertension. *Image: Journal of Nursing Scholarship*, 25(3), 204-207.

Kondora, L. L. (1993). A Heideggerian hermeneutical analysis of survivors of incest. *Image: Journal of Nursing Scholarship*, 25(1), 11-16.

Ragsdale, D., Kotarba, J. A., and Morrow, J. R. (1992). Quality of life of hospitalized persons with AIDS. *Image: Journal of Nursing Scholarship*, 24(4), 259-265.

Sayles-Cross, S. (1993). Perceptions of familial caregivers of elder adults. *Image: Journal of Nursing Scholarship*, 25(2), 88-92.

CHAPTER

15

Reliability and Validity

INTRODUCTION

The reliability and validity of the data collection instruments must be sound in order to have any confidence in the results. Any consumer of research must be able to critique the validity and reliability of instruments used in a research study. During the conduct of research, the possibility of systematic and random error must be kept at a minimum in order to believe the results of the study.

LEARNING OBJECTIVES

On completion of this chapter, the student should be able to do the following:

- Discuss reliability and validity as they relate to data collection instruments.
- Compare content, criterion, and construct validity in the choice of instruments used in research.
- Compare stability, homogeneity, and equivalence in determining reliability.
- Critique the validity and reliability reported in research studies.

ACTIVITY 1

Random or systematic error may occur in any research study. Identify the type of measurement error and how the error might have been reduced in the following examples.

1. A researcher noted that several subjects appeared nervous when asked to complete a questionnaire about anxiety.

   _____

   _____

2. It was discovered at the conclusion of a study that the scale was inaccurate by 5 pounds.

   _____

   _____

3. The research assistants did not receive any training or use a protocol prior to conducting the interviews.

_____

_____

Check your answers with those in Appendix A, Chapter 15.

ACTIVITY 2

Validity is the concern whether the measurement tools are actually measuring what they are supposed to measure. There are three basic concerns for measurement validity: content, criterion, and construct validity.

1. Content validity ascertains that the instrument is measuring within the domain of the construct intended to be measured. How might a researcher establish content validity of a new rating scale for maternal attachment?

_____

_____

2. Criterion validity examines whether the results of the measure are consistent with actual behavior. In this category are concurrent validity and predictive validity. A researcher wants to study how a patient's confidence in giving insulin injections affects his or her ability to self-administer insulin. How could the researcher establish the two types of criterion validity on a new measure of confidence?

_____

_____

3. Construct validity examines the extent that the test measures the phenomenon intended to be measured. Explain how you might examine convergent and divergent validity in developing a measure of social support.

_____

_____

4. If you believed your social support instrument measured two types of support, what would you expect to find in a factor analysis of the results from your instrument?

_____

_____

Check your answers with those in Appendix A, Chapter 15.

ACTIVITY 3

An instrument is considered reliable if it is accurate and consistent. If the concept being stud-ied is stable, the same results should occur when measurement is repeated. Reliability in-cludes the concepts of stability, homogeneity, and equivalence.

1. Give an example of each of the two types of tests for stability.

   _____

   _____

2. In what instance would it be better to use an alternate form rather than a test-retest measure for stability?

   _____

   _____

3. Homogeneity is a measure of internal consistency. All items on the instrument should be complementary and measure the same characteristic or concept. For each of the following examples, identify which type of test for homogeneity is described.

   a. The odd items of the test had a high correlation with the even numbers of the test.

   _____

   b. Each item on the test using a 5-point Likert scale had a moderate correlation with every other item on the test.

   _____

   c. Each item on the test ranged in correlation from .62 to .89 with the total.

   _____

   d. Each item on the true-false test had a moderate correlation with every other item on the test.

   _____

4. Equivalence means that the test is reliable and consistent. Two types of equivalence reported are parallel or alternate forms and interrater reliability. Complete the following sentence related to equivalence.

Four research assistants received training in how to categorize statements made from

transcripts of interviews. To establish _____ reliability, they individually analyzed and categorized the same set of transcripts and the results were compared, with an average correlation coefficient of .92 for 5 tapes.

Check your answers with those in Appendix A, Chapter 15.

ACTIVITY 4

Using the criteria listed in Chapter 15 in the text, critique the study by Stewart Fahs and Kinney (1991) found in the appendix of the text in terms of how well the researchers provided you with instrument reliability and validity information.

_____

_____

_____

_____

_____

_____

_____

_____

_____

_____

_____

_____

_____

_____

Check your answers with those in Appendix A, Chapter 15.

POSTTEST

Using the following terms, complete the sentences for the type of validity or reliability discussed.

content validity	test-retest reliability
factor analysis	Cronbach's alpha
convergent validity	alternate or parallel form
divergent validity	interrater reliability

1. In tests for reliability, the self-efficacy scale had a _____

   _____ of .88, demonstrating internal consistency for the new measure.

2. The ABC coping scale demonstrated _____ validity with

   correlation of .78 with the XYZ coping scale. _____
   validity was supported with correlation of .48 with the QRS stress scale.

3. The investigator established _____ validity through evaluation of the cardiac recovery scale by a panel of cardiac clinical nurse specialists. All items were rated 0 to 5 for importance to recovery and only items scoring above an average of 3 were kept in the final scale.

4. The results of the _____
   were that all the items clustered around three factors, lending support to the notion that there are three dimensions of coping.

5. The observations were rated by three experts. The _____
   reliability among the observers was 94%.

6. To assess _____ reliability, subjects completed the locus of control questionnaire at the beginning of the project and two weeks later. The correlation of .86 supports the stability of the concept of hardiness.

The answers to the posttest are in the Instructor's Resource Manual. Please check with your instructor for these answers.

REFERENCE

Stewart Fahs, P. S. and Kinney, M. R. (1991). The abdomen, thigh, and arm as sites for subcutaneous sodium heparin injections. *Nursing Research,* 40(4), 204-207.

16

Descriptive Data Analysis

INTRODUCTION

The concept of measurement forms an important link between the data collection and the data analysis components of a study. The researcher begins thinking about measurement when formulating the operational definitions of crucial variables. These operational definitions point to relevant data collection instruments. The choice of data analysis strategies is tied to the kinds of data collected and the level of measurement used with each method of data collection. The first few exercises in this chapter will focus on measurement.

Once you have reviewed the levels of measurement, the exercises will address descriptive data analysis strategies. The basic goal in the use of descriptive statistics is to provide the clearest possible summary of the sample data. Your task as a critical reader of research is to decide whether or not the statistics used are accurate, appropriate, and clearly presented.

LEARNING OBJECTIVES

On completion of this chapter, the student should be able to do the following:

- Distinguish among the four levels of measurement.
- Identify the level of measurement used in specified sets of data.
- Recognize the symbols associated with each of the descriptive statistical tools.
- Interpret accurately measures of central tendency and measures of variation.
- Critique the use of descriptive statistics in specified studies.

ACTIVITY 1

1. Match the level of measurement found in Column B with the appropriate example(s) in Column A. Some terms from Column B will be used more than once.

	Column A	Column B
1. _A_	method of birth control	a. nominal
A 2. _B_	light smokers vs. heavy smokers	b. ordinal
3. _D_	blood levels of catecholamines	c. interval
B 4. _C_	attitude toward family planning using 5-point Likert scale	d. ratio
5. _B_	quality of nursing care	
B 6. _C_	degree of depression	

7. C height and weight
8. B birth order
9. D pulse rate
10. B level of RN job satisfaction
11. C body temperature measured
with Centigrade thermometer
12. B systolic blood pressure

2. Read the following excerpts from specific studies. Identify the variable (or variables) and indicate which level of measurement would apply.

a. Each subject was randomly assigned to one of three treatment levels of oxygen flow (2, 4, 6 LPM) or to control. (Lim-Levy, 1982)

Name of variable _O2 flow._

Level of measurement _ratio_

b. Behavioral states of sleep (deep, light, drowsy) and awake (alert, active, crying) were assessed according to the Brazelton Neonatal Assessment Scale. (Franck, 1986)

Name of variable _states of sleep & awake._

Level of measurement _ordinal nominal_

c. The Revised UCLA Loneliness Scale is a 20-item Likert scale that measures the subjective experience of loneliness. . . . Scores on the 4-point scale can range from 20 to 80; the higher the score, the higher the loneliness. (Mahon and Yarcheski, 1992)

Name of variable _loneliness_

Level of measurement _interval_

d. An IVAC811 was used to measure the temperatures. The thermometer accuracy of ±0.02 degrees Fahrenheit meets U.S. government regulations for thermometers with a display registry of ±0.2 degrees Fahrenheit of a known temperature. (Hasler and Cohen, 1982)

Name of variable _temp._

Level of measurement _interval_

e. The Katz Index of Activities of Daily Living (ADL), used to assess functional status, measures levels of independence (graded in 6 categories) in performing six activities: bathing, dressing, toileting, transferring, continence, and feeding. . . . (Wanich, Sullivan-Marx, Gottlieb, and Johnson, 1992)

Name of variable _functional status_

Level of measurement ___nominal___

Knowledge of a given variable and the sophistication of available measuring (data collection) instruments influence the levels of measurement that exist in any given study. The level of measurement also points to the type of statistics used in the analysis of these data. Nonparametric statistics are used when data are at the nominal or ordinal level of measurement, while parametric statistics can be used with interval or ratio data. Parametric statistical tools are more powerful than nonparametric statistical tools.

3. Read the following example and answer the questions that follow.

A researcher is measuring the amount of pain associated with two different ways of completing a particular procedure. Specific indicators of several levels of pain are defined, so the observer marks the appropriate spot on the rating scale at various intervals during the procedure. The rating scale looks like this:

0	1	2	3	4	5
no pain	minimal pain	some pain	moderate pain	considerable pain	intolerable pain

Data indicating the amount of observed pain experience of one client undergoing each of the two procedures is given below.

Observation	Procedure 1, Client 1	Procedure 2, Client 1
1	4.6	1.8
2	3.2	1.1
3	1.9	4.8
4	4.5	2.8
5	3.3	3.2

a. What level of measurement is being used? Explain your answer.

_____

b. Which type of statistics (parametric or nonparametric) would be appropriate to choose in an analysis of these data?

_____

When critiquing a study that uses a scale like the one in #3, one must walk softly. If you, the reader, adhere strictly to the categories of measurement and view the data as ordinal, but the researcher treated the data as interval, then you will be inclined to criticize heavily those studies that mismatch the type of measured data and the analysis strategies. But if you, the reader, recognize how widespread the practice of treating ordinal as interval data is and ignore the mismatches when they occur, bad habits are perpetuated. A useful middle road in critiquing is to point out the mismatch but not to do so vehemently. With that in mind, move on to Activity 2.

Check your answers with those in Appendix A, Chapter 16.

ACTIVITY 2

1. A brief review of some aspects of descriptive statistics will establish some common ground before you practice the interpretation and critiquing of descriptive statistics. Decide which of the items listed below is related to a measure of central tendency and which to a measure of variation. Use the abbreviations from the key provided.

    KEY: CT = measure of central tendency
              V = measure of variation

    a. _CT_ X
    b. _V_ Range
    c. _CT_ Mode
    d. _V_ S
    e. _CT_ S.D.
    f. _CT_ Media
    g. _CT_ Mean

2. Each item on the following list is a dependent variable from an actual piece of research. Identify which level of measurement is being used. Identify which measure of central tendency and which measure of variation would be appropriate.

    a. Client's distress (e.g., pain, discomfort, and anxiety) on a scale with 1 meaning no distress and 15 meaning extreme distress.

    Level of measurement _Ordinal_ Central tendency _____ Variation _____

    b. Functioning of single parents established by two out of three professionals independently deciding whether observed parenting behavior in several categories was adequate or not.

    Level of measurement _____ Central tendency _____ Variation _____

    c. Sucking response of newborns measured using a suckometer/research nipple that records sucking pressure in mmHg.

    Level of measurement _interval_ Central tendency _____ Variation _____

    d. Number of medication errors occurring in a 24-hour period.

    Level of measurement _ratio_ Central tendency _____ Variation _____

    e. Skewed distribution of income.

    Level of measurement _ratio_ Central tendency _____ Variation _____

Check your answers with those in Appendix A, Chapter 16.

ACTIVITY 3

Activity 2 provided you with practice in finding the descriptive statistics in a study. The next task is the initial interpretation and critique of the use of these statistics.

1. Table 1 from the Hartfield, Cason, and Cason (1983) study is duplicated below. Use the data in the table to answer the questions.

TABLE 1
Means and Standard Deviations for State, Trait and Sensation Scores by Information Group

	Sensation		Procedure	
Information Groups (N = 10)				
	$\bar{x}$	S.D.	$\bar{x}$	S.D.
Anxiety scores				
State	39.9	12.41	50.8	12.07
Trait	35.7	6.78	35.6	7.71
Sensation scores				
Preinformation	35.7	7.54	32.9	8.62
Postinformation	42.0	8.89	31.6	8.82
Postprocedure	45.8	9.60	45.1	9.80

a. What is the highest mean reported? _____

b. For what group and what variable is the highest mean reported?

Group _____

Variable _____

c. Which group of sensation scores is the most homogeneous (i.e., has the least variation)?

_____

d. Following is the text in which the researchers discuss the data in Table 1 above. Determine whether the information in the table and the information in the text agree. (Note: Don't worry about the $p < .05$ or $p > .05$ notations.)

"For the group that had received sensation information, the mean score on the sensation inventory postinformation and preprocedure was not significantly different ($d = 3.8$; $p > .05$) from the sensation inventory score obtained postprocedure. On average there was congruence between the responses the sensation information group reported as expected (once information had been given them) and what was reported as experienced.

By contrast, those in the procedural information group had mean sensation inventory scores postinformation and preprocedure which were statistically different (d = 12.1; p < .05) from the mean postprocedure scores. On average there was a lack of congruence between what was reported as expected and what was subsequently reported as experienced by persons in the procedural information group." (Hartfield, Cason, and Cason, 1982)

Do the information in the table and the information in the text agree? Yes No

e. Given the title of the study and the information in Table 1 and its accompanying text, what inferences would you expect the researchers to draw?

_____

_____

_____

Check your answers with those in Appendix A, Chapter 16.

2. Table 2 from the Keane, Ducette, and Adler study is duplicated below. Use the data in the table to answer the questions.

TABLE 2
Means and Standards Deviations of the Staff Burnout Scale for Health Professionals by Unit

	Surgical ICU	Medical ICU	Intermediate Surgical	Intermediate Medical	General Surgical	General Medical	Total
$\bar{x}$	49.9	51.2	57.3	46.4	43.9	65.2	52.1
S.D.	14.3	13.4	14.9	14.7	16.5	20.5	15.6

a. The nurses from which unit had the highest mean burnout score? _____

b. What was the standard deviation for the group with the highest burnout score?

_____

c. What is the relationship between the standard deviation of the group of nurses with the highest burnout score and the standard deviations of the other groups?

_____

_____

d. What does this tell you about the group with the highest burnout scores?

_____

_____

e. Given the information in the answers to the previous four questions, what conclusions would you draw about the nurses on the general medical unit used in this study?

_____

_____

_____

_____

3. Provide the answers requested in each item.

a. Two outpatient clinics measured client waiting time as one indicator of effectiveness. The mean and standard deviation of waiting time in minutes is reported below. Which outpatient clinic would you prefer, assuming that all other things are equal? Explain your answer.

	Clinic 1	Clinic 2
Mean (in minutes)	40	25
Standard deviation (in minutes)	10	45

_____

_____

_____

_____

b. You are responsible for ordering urinary catheters for your unit. Which measure of central tendency would be the most useful?

_____

c. Below are two histograms. Which group has the biggest standard deviation?

_____

_____

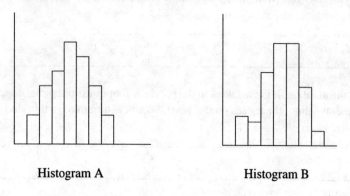

Histogram A   Histogram B

Check your answers with those in Appendix A, Chapter 16.

POSTTEST

Study 1

Use data from the following table to answer the questions that follow.

TABLE 3
Mean Scores on Sex Knowledge Test of Adolescents Rated as Effective or Ineffective in Contraceptive Use

Time of Counseling	Effective Users			Ineffective Users			Total		
	$\bar{x}$	S.D.	N	$\bar{x}$	S.D.	N	$\bar{x}$	S.D.	N
Negative pregnancy test	28.35	4.39	26	29.00	5.70	9	28.51	4.68	35
Routine medical visit	26.33	6.86	33	19.30	6.86	10	24.70	7.42	43
Total	27.22	5.94	59	23.89	7.92	19	26.41	6.58	78

Source: March, S. A., Brown, J. S., and Danielson, R. (1983). Contraceptive use by adolescent females in relation to knowledge and to time and method of contraceptive counseling, *Research in Nursing and Health*, 6(4), 175-182.

1. What was the total number of adolescents counseled at the time they received the results

   of a negative pregnancy test? _____

2. How many adolescents participated in the study? _____

3. Which group had the highest score on the Sex Knowledge Test? _____

4. Which group showed the least amount of variation in scores on the Sex Knowledge Test?

   _____

5. Based on the data presented in this table, respond to the following statements. Use the abbreviations from the key provided.

   KEY: T = true
         F = false
         ? = unable to determine

   a. _____ The amount of knowledge about sex is not a critical factor in determining effective use of contraceptives.
   b. _____ Forty-two percent of the adolescents were effective users of contraceptives.
   c. _____ A score of 29.00 on the Sex Knowledge Test indicates a large amount of knowledge.
   d. _____ A larger number of effective users of contraceptives were counseled during a routine medical visit than when receiving the results of a negative pregnancy test.
   e. _____ Adolescents counseled at the time of receiving a negative pregnancy test are more alike in Sex Knowledge Test scores than those who received counseling during a routine medical visit.
   f. _____ Sex education is futile.

Study 2

Critique the following excerpt and table from a fictitious study:

Three hundred sixty-one adults constituted the study sample; 133 were males and 228 were females. Subjects ranged in age from 20 to 88 years. The mean age of the sample was 63 with a standard deviation of 11.60, and the median age was 55. Of the respondents, 53% (191) were married, 19% (69) were widowed, 11% (40) were divorced, and 8% (29) were single. The rest were either separated, engaged, or living as married.

TABLE 4
Marital Status of the Bereaved and Control Group as Percentage of Total

	Bereaved	Control	Total
Married	84 (24%)	104 (29%)	191
Widowed	45 (13%)	24 (7%)	69
Divorced	16 (4%)	24 (7%)	40
Single	9 (2%)	20 (6%)	29
Other	11 (3%)	20 (6%)	32
Totals	168 (47%)	193 (53%)	361 (100%)

_____

_____

_____

_____

_____

The answers to the posttest are in the Instructor's Resource Manual. Please check with your instructor for these answers.

REFERENCES

Hartfield, M. T., Cason, C. L., and Cason, G. J. (1983). Effects of information about a threatening procedure on patients' expectations and emotional distress. *Nursing Research,* 31(4), 202-206.

Keane, A., Ducette, J., and Adler, D. C. (1985). Stress in ICU and non-ICU nurses. *Nursing Research,* 34(4), 231-236.

Mahon, N. E. and Yarcheski, A. (1992). Alternate explanations of loneliness in adolescents: A replication and extension study. *Nursing Research,* 41(3), 151-156.

March, S. A., Brown, J. S., and Danielson, R. (1983). Contraceptive use by adolescent females in relation to knowledge and to time and method of contraceptive counseling. *Research in Nursing and Health,* 6(4), 175-182.

CHAPTER

17

Inferential Data Analysis

INTRODUCTION

Chapter 16 introduced you to descriptive data analysis. Descriptive statistics are very valuable in situations where the researcher's interest does not go beyond the group of people or data that is immediately available. Frequently the researcher is more interested in using the information from the sample to learn about the population. To do so, the researcher needs to employ different research designs and analyze the data with the tools of inferential statistics. This chapter provides you with opportunities to think through the logic leading to the use of inferential statistics.

Please note that some of the studies used in this chapter are dated. They continue to be used because they provide good examples of the application of statistical strategies.

LEARNING OBJECTIVES

On completion of this chapter, the student should be able to do the following:

- Identify the symbols representing specified inferential statistical techniques.
- State the null hypothesis given a research hypothesis.
- Choose an appropriate inferential statistical strategy for specified research hypotheses.
- Think through the process of hypothesis testing.
- Interpret the results of specified inferential statistical tests.
- Critique the use of inferential statistics in given studies.

ACTIVITY 1

In each of the following sets, match the item in Column B with the term in Column A. In Sets 2 and 3, the items in Column B will be used more than once.

Column A | Column B

Set 1
1. _____ analysis of variance   a. r
2. _____ Pearson correlation coefficient   b. F
3. _____ chi-square   c. X^2
4. _____ student's t-test   d. t

Set 2

1. _____ ANOVA   a. appropriate for two groups
2. _____ X^2 b. appropriate for three or more groups
3. _____ t-test
4. _____ Kruskal-Wallis (H)

Set 3

1. _____ t   a. parametric
2. _____ X^2 b. nonparametric
3. _____ r (Pearson)
4. _____ F
5. _____ U
6. _____ H
7. _____ r (Spearman)

Check your answers with those in Appendix A, Chapter 17.

ACTIVITY 2

For the following research hypotheses, state the null hypothesis.

1. "It was hypothesized that among female cholecystectomy patients, preoperative self-efficacy would be related positively to postoperative ambulation, deep breathing, recall of expected events, and requests for pain medication." (Oetker-Black, Hart, Hoffman, and Geary, 1992)

   _____

   _____

   _____

2. "Hypertensive clients will report lower levels of total sexual functioning than nonhypertensive clients." (Watts, 1982)

   _____

   _____

   _____

3. "There is a difference between runners and nonrunners in the relative value placed on personal health." (Walsh, 1985)

   _____

   _____

   _____

Check your answers with those in Appendix A, Chapter 17.

ACTIVITY 3

Choosing which inferential statistic to use in testing for a specific hypothesis consists of a chain of decisions. You can use that same chain of decisions as a critiquing tool. Given one hypothesis and a list of the critical questions, you and the researcher should come to the same conclusion as to which inferential strategy was appropriate. If your conclusions are different (e.g., you use a t-test and the researcher used ANOVA), something is wrong. You then have the task of discovering who goofed.

Now for some practice. You will be using Figure 1 on the next page to answer questions regarding the hypotheses that follow. One sample hypothesis has been worked through. You need to apply the same process to hypotheses 2 through 4.

First, consider the critical questions:

1. Does the hypothesis address differences or associations?
2. Which level of measurement was used in measuring the dependent variable?
3. How many groups exist?
4. Are the groups independent or dependent?
5. What are your conclusions? What would be an appropriate statistical strategy?

Second, look over Figure 1. Then read the four hypotheses and follow the process through the diagram in Figure 1.

Hypothesis 1

"There is a difference in the number of microorganisms present on hands wearing rings compared to hands not wearing rings." (Jacobson, Thiele, McCune, and Farrell, 1985)

Critical Questions

1. Does the hypothesis address differences or associations?

   The hypothesis clearly states, "There is a difference . . .."

2. Which level of measurement was used in measuring the dependent variable?

   The dependent variable is the number of microorganisms, and microorganisms usually are measured in number per some standard measure; therefore, I would say ratio level of measurement. Just to be sure, I would check the methodology part of the study to see the exact procedure used.

3. How many groups exist?

   Two: microorganisms from hands with rings and from hands without rings.

4. Are the groups independent or dependent?

Dependent. Each pair of hands was tested under both conditions (with rings and without rings). So subject 1 wore rings for several days and then went to the lab and followed the handwashing procedure. Then subject 1 took off all rings for several days, went to the lab, and followed the handwashing procedure. This allowed the researchers to control for a variety of factors that could have produced error.

5. Conclusion:

Data should have been analyzed using the paired (or dependent) t-test. They were as the quote from the study indicates: "Paired t-tests were used to compare each subject's before and after scrubbing platings (see Table 1)."

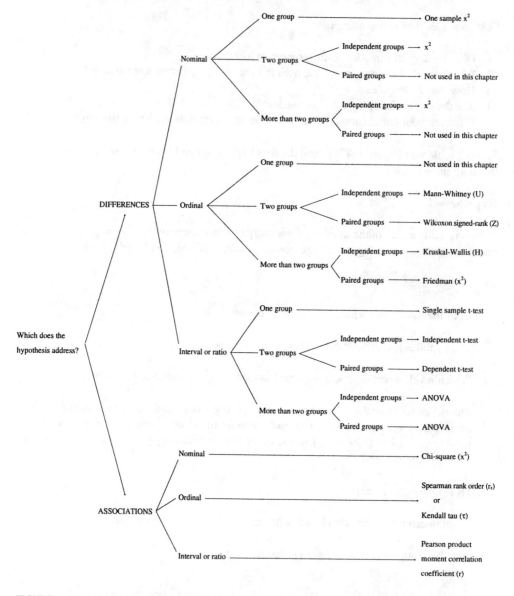

FIGURE 1. Adapted from Knapp, R. G. (1985). *Basic statistics for nurses*, 2d ed., New York, Wiley.

Hypothesis 2

"There is no relationship between axillary and rectal temperatures in the normal full-term neonate." (Schiffman, 1982)

Critical Questions

1. Does the hypothesis address differences or associations?

_____

2. The dependent variable is:

   a. neonate
   b. axillary temperature
   c. temperature

3. The level of measurement used for the dependent variable is:

   a. nominal
   b. ordinal
   c. interval
   d. ratio
   e. need more information

4. Which of the following tests of association would be appropriate?

   a. Chi-square
   b. Spearman rank order
   c. Kendall tau
   d. Pearson product moment correlation coefficient

Hypothesis 3

"The dominant concerns expressed by preschool healthy children, acutely ill children, chronically ill children in short-stay hospitalizations, and chronically ill children in long-stay hospitalizations are different." (Ritchie, Caty, and Ellerton, 1984)

Critical Questions

1. This hypothesis addressed:

   a. an association
   b. differences

2. The independent variable is:

   a. age of children
   b. health status of children

c. concerns of the parents of ill children
d. effects of hospitalization on children

3. The dependent variable is:

   a. hospitalization versus nonhospitalization
   b. health status of children
   c. the expressed concerns of children
   d. differences in hospital lengths of stay

4. The dependent variable is measured on which of the following scales?

   a. nominal
   b. ordinal
   c. interval
   d. ratio
   e. need more information

5. The number of groups from which data were collected is:

   a. 4
   b. 3
   c. 2
   d. 1

6. Were the groups independent or dependent? _____

7. Which of the following tests could be appropriate?

   a. t-test
   b. Mann-Whitney (U)
   c. Kruskal-Wallis (H)
   d. ANOVA (F)

Now you do one using just the critical questions as a guide.

Hypothesis 4

"After treatment, the group receiving a towel bath will have lower post-treatment anxiety scores than patients receiving a conventional bed bath." (Barsevick and Llewellyn, 1982)

Critical Questions

1. Differences or associations? _____

2. Dependent variable and its level of measurement?

   _____

3. Number of groups? _____

4. Groups independent or independent? _____

5. Appropriate statistical strategy? _____

Check your answers with those in Appendix A, Chapter 17.

ACTIVITY 4

Once you have determined whether or not the correct test of statistical significance has been chosen, you need to be able to interpret the statistical significance decision reached using that particular test. Information you will need would be (a) knowledge of the symbols associated with each test; (b) the usual form used in writing the decisions; (c) introductory concepts of probability; and (d) the process of hypothesis testing. Given the amount of space available in a book devoted to the understanding of the research process, only the briefest of introductions can be provided. You are encouraged to consult your instructor, a statistics text, or a statistics class for more detailed explanations.

Chapter 17 in the text outlines the steps to hypothesis testing:

1. State the research hypothesis (H_R).
2. State the null hypothesis (H_O). Most researchers do not state the null hypothesis in a formal manner. They do know that this is the one being tested by the relevant test of statistical significance.
3. Set the level of acceptable probability. Frequently this value is at the .05 or .01 level in nursing research.
4. Collect data and compute the appropriate test of statistical significance.
5. Compare the number obtained at the end of those computations with the established table value. If the number from the data in this study is less than that in the table, then statistical significance has not been reached. If the number from the data in the study is greater than the number in the table, then statistical significance has been reached.
6. If statistical significance was not reached, one must support the null hypothesis and, by inference, be unable to support the research hypothesis. If statistical significance was reached, one rejects the null hypothesis and, by inference, supports the research hypothesis.

Again, let's walk through an example and then you can practice with additional examples. We'll use the first hypothesis discussed in Activity 3: handwashing, microorganisms, and rings on hands.

1. State the research hypothesis.

   There is a difference in the number of microorganisms on hands wearing rings when compared with hands not wearing rings.

2. State the null hypothesis.

There is no difference in the number of microorganisms between hands wearing rings and hands not wearing rings.

3. Set the level of acceptable probability.

It is $p = .05$, which means that a difference between the microorganism count between the hands with rings and the hands without had to have occurred no more than 5 times out of 100 replications of this experiment.

4. Collect data and compute the appropriate test of statistical significance.
   See the information below:

Sample

After handwashing	Mean	S.D.		
No rings	1,597	2,346	}	Difference mean = -842
With rings	2,438	3,717	}	t-value = -1.13
			}	df = 31

5. Compare the number obtained at the end of those computations with the established table value.

Done. The t of -1.13 with 31 degrees of freedom was compared with the table value necessary to reach $p = .05$. The table value is 2.04 (it is unnecessary to pay attention to the negative and positive signs in this situation). The number from the study's data is smaller than the respective table value, so statistical significance was not reached.

6. Statistical significance was not reached, so the null hypothesis is accepted. We have no evidence to argue against the statement that there is no difference in the number of micro-organisms between hands wearing rings and hands not wearing rings. By inference, we cannot support the research hypothesis that there is a difference. Given the data from this study, the wearing of rings made no difference in the number of microorganisms after handwashing.

OK? Now it's your turn. Work through the same process. Ask and answer the same questions used above for the following hypothesis. You will have to make one exception to the above process. You will not be expected to determine the table value for the calculated test statistic. You will need to accept the values and decisions reported by the researchers.

Hypothesis 1

"There is a difference between runners and nonrunners in the relative value placed on personal health."

Reported data: "The first hypothesis, that there is a difference between runners and nonrunners in the relative value placed on personal health, was tested using the Mann-Whitney U, with alpha set at .05, and was accepted, $p < .019$. The value of U was found to be 1876.5; of U', 4990.5. Greater value was placed on personal health by the runners than by the nonrunners." (Walsh, 1985)

1. The research hypothesis is stated above. The null hypothesis would be: There is no difference between runners and nonrunners in the relative value placed on personal health.

2. What preset level of probability is stated as acceptable?

   _____

3. What level of probability was found to exist between the two sets of data?

   _____

4. Are these data statistically significant?

   _____

5. Was the null hypothesis accepted or rejected?

   _____

6. Was the research hypothesis supported or not supported (accepted or rejected)?

   _____

7. Write out the steps in your thinking that led you to the answer in #6.

   _____

   _____

   _____

Hypothesis 2

"After treatment, the group receiving a towel bath will have lower anxiety scores than patients receiving a conventional bed bath."

Reported data. "Two sample t-tests were used on the state anxiety scores and palmar sweat scores to test the hypothesis that patients receiving a towel bath will have lower anxiety scores than patients receiving a conventional bed bath. The conventional bath group and the towel bath group showed no significant differences in group means prior to the bath for either state anxiety or palmar sweating. Immediately after the bathing procedure, a significant difference in group means was observed for the STAI A-State subscale ($t = -2.04$, $p = 0.045$), with lower scores for patients receiving a towel bath. This difference was not noted one hour following the bath. At no time were there significant differences in palmar sweat scores." (Barsevick and Llewellyn, 1982)

1. The research hypothesis is stated. The null hypothesis would be:

   _____

2. What is the stated level of the preset acceptable degree of probability? (Careful, this one can be a bit tricky.)

_____

_____

3. What level of probability was found to exist between the towel-bathed and the conventionally-bathed groups?

_____

4. Is this value statistically significant?

_____

5. Was the null hypothesis accepted or rejected?

_____

6. Was the research hypothesis supported or not supported (accepted or rejected)?

_____

7. Write out the steps in your thinking that led you to the answer in #6.

_____

_____

_____

Check your answers with those in Appendix A, Chapter 17.

POSTTEST

Indicate whether the following values are statistically significant or not statistically significant. Use the abbreviations from the key provided.

KEY: A = statistically significant
         B = not statistically significant

1. _____ $X^2 = 13.07$, df = 2, p = .05. Critical table value is 5.99.
2. _____ t = 2.03, df = 38, p = .01. Critical table value is 2.42.
3. _____ t = 6.79, df = 58, p = .05. Critical table value is 1.67.
4. _____ F(3,16) = 19.20, p = .01. Critical table value is 5.29.
5. _____ F(2,20) = 2.67, p = .05. Critical table value is 3.49.

Use the following material from a study to answer questions 6 through 15.

One important way in which people perceive events is in terms of the degree to which they believe they have influence over the outcome of an event, which has been called locus of control . . . results suggest that personal control can reduce the aversiveness of a noxious stimulus and increase performance and information seeking. Events perceived as uncontrollable (external locus of control) lead to response behaviors such as helplessness, reduced acquisition of information and detachment from the stressful stimuli (p.76). The hypothesis tested in this study was that degree of internality on the Nowicki-Strickland Locus of Control Scale for Children and active coping will be related (p.77). A Pearson correlational analysis evidenced a significant inverse relationship between locus of control and avoidant-active coping ($r = -0.39$, $p < .01$). This indicates active coping is significantly associated with internal locus of control. To clarify this relationship, an analysis of variance showed a significant difference ($F(2,48) = 3.59$, $p < .05$) between coping groups on locus of control score. This analysis is summarized in Table 1.

TABLE 1

Summary of Analysis of Variance between Coping Groups on Locus of Control

			$\overline{M}$	S.D.
Avoidant			15.33	3.75
Middle			14.61	4.52
Active			11.00	4.05
Source	df	SS	MS	F
Between groups	2	130.66	65.33	3.60*
Within groups	48	871.34	18.15	

*$p < .05$.

Note: Higher scores indicate more external locus of control

Source: Lamontagene, L. L. (1984). Children's locus of control beliefs as predictors of preoperative coping behavior. *Nursing Research*, 33, 76-79, 85.

6. State the research hypothesis (H_R).

_____

7. State the null hypothesis (H_O).

_____

8. The use of a Pearson correlation coefficient and analysis of variance indicate that coping behavior was measured on:

   a. a nominal scale

   b. an ordinal scale

   c. an interval or ratio scale

9. What level of probability was used with the Pearson correlation coefficient?

   _____

10. What level of probability was used with the analysis of variance?

   _____

11. Were the results statistically significant?

   a. Pearson correlation coefficient   Yes   No
   b. Analysis of variance   Yes   No

12. Which of the coping groups had the highest locus of control scores?

   _____

13. Which of the coping groups showed the most variation in locus of control scores?

   _____

14. Based on the analysis, which of the following was possible? Choose two:

   a. Accept the null hypothesis.
   b. Reject the null hypothesis.
   c. Support the research hypothesis.
   d. Do not support the research hypothesis.

15. Explain the following sentence: "The results were statistically significant at the .05 level of probability."

   _____

   _____

   _____

   _____

   _____

The answers to the posttest are in the Instructor's Resource Manual. Please check with your instructor for these answers.

REFERENCES

Oetker-Black, S. L., Hart, F., Hoffman, J., and Geary, S. (1992). Preoperative self-efficacy and postoperative behaviors. *Applied Nursing Research, 5*(3), 134-139.

Barsevick, A. and Llewellyn, J. (1982). A comparison of the anxiety-reducing potential of two techniques of bathing. *Nursing Research,* 31(1), 17-22.

Jacobson, G., Thiele, J. E., McCune, J. H., and Farrel, L. D. (1985). Handwashing: Ring-wearing and number of microorganisms. *Nursing Research,* 34(3), 186-188.

Knapp, R. G. (1985). *Basic statistics for nurses.* 2nd ed., New York, NY, Wiley.

Lamontagene, L. L. (1984). Children's locus of control beliefs as predictors of preoperative coping behavior. *Nursing Research,* 33, 76-79, 85.

Ritchie, J. A., Caty, S., and Ellerton, M. L. (1984). Concerns of acutely ill, chronically ill, and healthy preschool children. *Research in Nursing and Health,* 7, 265-274.

Schiffman, R. F. (1982). Temperature monitoring in the neonate: A comparison of axillary and rectal temperatures. *Nursing Research,* 31(5), 274-277.

Walsh, V. R. (1985). Health beliefs and practices of runners versus nonrunners. *Nursing Research, 34(6),* 353-356.

Watts, R. J. (1982). Sexual functioning, health beliefs, and compliance with high blood pressure medications. *Nursing Research,* 31(5), 278-283.

18

Analysis of the Findings

INTRODUCTION

As the last sections of a research report, the results and conclusions sections answer the question "so what?" In other words, it is in these two sections the investigator "makes sense" of the research, critically synthesizes the data, applies them (or ties them) to a theoretical framework, and builds on a body of knowledge. These two sections then become a most important part of the research report because they describe the generalizability of the findings and offer recommendations for further research.

Well-written, clear, and concise results and conclusions sections provide valuable information for nursing practice. Conversely, poorly written sections leave the critiquer bewildered, confused, and wondering how or if the findings are relevant to nursing.

LEARNING OBJECTIVES

On completion of this chapter, the student should be able to do the following:

- Know the difference between the results sections of a study and the discussion sections of the study.
- Interpret table and figure findings from a research report.
- Describe various generalizations and limitations of a research report.
- Identify recommendations from a research report.

ACTIVITY 1

Knowing what information to look for and where to find it in the results and discussions sections of a research report will enable you to interpret the research findings and critique research reports.

1. Identify the section in which the following information from the research report may be found. Put an **A** if the information can be found in the results section and a **B** if the information can be found in the discussion section.

   a. _____ Tables/figures
   b. _____ Limitations of the study
   c. _____ Relates data analysis to the literature review
   d. _____ Makes inferences (generalizes results)
   e. _____ Hypotheses supported/non-supported statistically

f. _____ Hypotheses test findings

g. _____ Statistical tests used to analyze hypotheses

h. _____ Applies meaning (makes sense) of data analysis

i. _____ Suggests further research

j. _____ Suggests recommendations for nursing practice

2. Read the results and discussion section of the study "The Abdomen, Thigh, and Arm as Sites for Subcutaneous Sodium Heparin Injections" by Stewart Fahs and Kinney (1991) found in Appendix A of the text, and answer the following questions:

a. Low-dose heparin therapy does not differ in effectiveness when administered in the abdomen, thigh, or arm.
Yes No

b. More bruising occurred on subjects' thighs than on abdomens or arms.
Yes No

c. Larger bruises occurred on subjects' abdomen than on thighs or arms.
Yes No

d. The results from the study indicate that bruising occurred in 89% of all the 299 injections.
Yes No

e. It is recommended that low-dose heparin injections be given subcutaneously in the thigh in order for the medication to be most effective and cause least bruising.
Yes No

f. Future studies should consider measuring bruising produced by subcutaneous heparin injections 60-72 hours after the injection is given.
Yes No

g. The study found that subjects greatly feared getting an injection in the abdomen.
Yes No

h. The practice of giving low-dose heparin therapy solely in the abdomen was not supported in this study.
Yes No

i. The authors suggest further studies should involve evaluating patients' physical and emotional discomfort experienced when receiving low-dose heparin therapy.
Yes No

j. Race accounted for differences in bruising among the subjects in the study.
Yes No

3. Discuss how the results of the Stewart Fahs and Kinney study could change your nursing practice in giving low-dose heparin therapy. After reading the results and discussion sections of the article, state 3-5 interventions you might consider doing differently in giving low-dose heparin.

_____

_____

_____

_____

_____

4. If you were a nurse manager, state ways you could disseminate the Stewart Fahs and Kinney findings to other staff members.

_____

_____

_____

_____

_____

_____

Check your answers with those in Appendix A, Chapter 18.

ACTIVITY 2

Being able to interpret and evaluate research report tables and figures enables you to gain a full picture of the research results.

1. Using the Stewart Fahs and Kinney (1991) article found in Appendix A of the text, refer to Tables 1, 2, and 3 found in the results section of the article. Answer the following questions related to the three tables.

a. The abbreviation ANOVA in Table 3 title is not spelled out in the article.
   Yes No

b. Table 3 indicates sample size for the study.
   Yes No

c. The variable being compared in Table 3 is surface areas of bruising on subjects' abdomen, thigh, and arm.
   Yes No

d. The probability level (p > .05) on Table 3 is in error. It should read (p < .05).
Yes No

e. According to Table 3, there is a difference in bruise size among the three injection sites 48 hours after the injections were administered.
Yes No

f. In Table 1, how many injections were administered to the subjects in the study?
a. 101   b. 97   c. 202   d. 299

g. Table 1 indicates that the fewest bruises occurred during injection:
a. 1   b. 2   c. 3

h. Table 1 indicates fewest bruises occurred in which site?
a. abdomen   b. thigh   c. arm

i. In Table 1, for all 3 injections and all 3 sites, how many total injections produced no bruising?
a. 20   b. 30   c. 40   d. 50

j. In Table 2, the greatest mean surface area of bruising on the arm occurred how many hours postinjection?
a. 48   b. 60   c. 72   d. unknown

2. Rewrite the title for Table 3 to more accurately reflect what the table is describing.

_____

3. Review the criteria of a "good" table. Analyze Table 3 and make 3-4 suggestions for change.

_____

_____

_____

Check your answers with those in Appendix A, Chapter 18.

ACTIVITY 3

Being able to interpret the findings and identify generalizations and limitations of research reports enables you to build on your personal body of knowledge and inform other members of your profession about new knowledge.

Read the article "Coping and Adaptation in Children with Diabetes" by Grey, Cameron, and Thurber (1991) found in Appendix B of the text.

1. After reading the discussion section, list 6-8 generalizations the authors make from the study's results.

   _____

   _____

   _____

   _____

   _____

2. Identify 2-3 limitations (weaknesses) of the study described by the authors and ones you may have found.

   _____

   _____

   _____

   _____

3. You are a nurse caring for a 12-year-old boy who has been newly diagnosed with insulin dependent diabetes. From the results discussed in Grey's, Cameron's, and Thurber's article, describe how you may expect him to "deal" with his diagnosis.

   _____

   _____

   _____

   _____

4. Describe strategies you may use to help this 12-year-old deal with the diabetes. What would you do for both the boy and his parents to help them adjust to his having diabetes?

   _____

   _____

   _____

   _____

Check your answers with those in Appendix A, Chapter 18.

ACTIVITY 4

Interpreting recommendations the investigators make from the research report findings enables you to pursue further research and make changes in your nursing practice.

Read the discussion section in the article "Types and Meanings of Caring Behaviors Among Elderly Nursing Home Residents" by Hutchison and Bahr (1991) found in Appendix C of the text.

1. List 4-5 recommendations the authors make that may be used in working with and caring for the elderly nursing home residents.

   _____

   _____

   _____

   _____

2. Based on the recommendations from Hutchison's and Bahr's article and assuming you are a staff nurse employed in a nursing home, devise a list of "daily" activities that nursing home residents could do to "care" for other residents in the nursing home.

   Example - Read a book to one of the residents who has poor eyesight.

   _____

   _____

   _____

   _____

Check your answers with those in Appendix A, Chapter 18.

POSTTEST

1. When a research hypothesis is supported through testing, it may be assumed that the hypothesis was:

   a. proved
   b. accepted
   c. rejected
   d. disconfirmed

2. True   False   Limitations of a study describe its weaknesses.

3. The results section of a research study includes all the following except:

    a. hypothesis testing results
    b. tables and figures
    c. statistical test description
    d. limitations of the study

4. True   False   Unsupported hypotheses mean that the study is of little value in generating knowledge.

5. Tables in research reports should meet all the following criteria except:

    a. clear, concise titles
    b. restate the text narrative
    c. economize the text
    d. supplement the text narrative

6. The discussion section provides opportunity for the investigator to do all the following except:

    a. describe implications from the research results
    b. relate the results to the literature review
    c. make generalizations to large populations of subjects
    d. suggest areas for further research

7. True   False   Hypothesis testing is described in the discussion section of the research report.

The answers to the posttest are in the Instructor's Resource Manual. Please check with your instructor for these answers.

REFERENCES

Grey, M., Cameron, M. E., and Thurber, F. W. (1991). Coping and adaptation in children with diabetes. *Nursing Research,* 40(3), 144-149.

Hutchison, C. P. and Bahr, R. T. (1991). Types and meanings of caring behaviors among elderly nursing home residents. *Image: Journal of Nursing Scholarship,* 23(2), 85-88.

Stewart Fahs, P. S. and Kinney, M. R. (1991). The abdomen, thigh, and arm as sites for subcutaneous sodium heparin injections. *Nursing Research,* 40(4), 204-207.

CHAPTER

19

Evaluating Quantitative Research

INTRODUCTION

Now that you have practiced analyzing each part of a research study, you are ready to put the complete critiquing process into practice. Critiquing entire studies takes some time initially, but the more you practice the easier it becomes.

LEARNING OBJECTIVES

On completion of this chapter, the student should be able to do the following:

- Identify journals with the primary focus of publishing reports of nursing research.
- Differentiate among stylistic considerations, scientific merit, and value to clinical practice relative to nursing research.
- List the content sections to be addressed when critiquing a research article.
- Critique a research article using the identified content sections.

ACTIVITY 1

1. In your role as a consumer of research, you will need to identify those nursing journals known to have the publishing of research as their primary publication goal. Indicate with a star (*) which of the following journals would likely focus on publishing research-based articles:

   a. _____ *Nursing Research*
   b. _____ *Image*
   c. _____ *Journal of Obstetric, Gynecologic, and Neonatal Nursing*
   d. _____ *Western Journal of Nursing Research*
   e. _____ *Nursing 93*
   f. _____ *American Journal of Nursing*
   g. _____ *RN*
   h. _____ *Applied Nursing Research*

2. Which of the research journals identified in item #1 are available in:

a. your school of nursing library?

_____

b. your general university library?

_____

c. the agency where you currently are in clinical practice (either for class or employment)?

_____

3. Name the four essential headings that would be found in published research studies.

a. _____

b. _____

c. _____

d. _____

Check your answers with those in Appendix A, Chapter 19.

ACTIVITY 2

Match the aspect of a reported research study in Column B with the descriptive phrase in Column A. Items in Column B will be used more than once.

Column A	Column B
1. _____ objective and unbiased	a. stylistic considerations
2. _____ expression of author's preference	b. scientific merit
3. _____ focuses on study's strengths and limitations	c. value of the study for
4. _____ considers cost and risks to clients	clinical practice
5. _____ requirements of a specific journal	
6. _____ addresses questions that begin with "should" or "can"	

Check your answers with those in Appendix A, Chapter 19.

ACTIVITY 3

List the content sections that have been identified throughout the text as important when critiquing a research article.

1. _____

2. _____

3. _____

4. _____

5. _____

6. _____

7. _____

8. _____

9. _____

10. _____

11. _____

12. _____

13. _____

14. _____

15. _____

16. _____

17. _____

Check your answers with those in Appendix A, Chapter 19.

ACTIVITY 4

Read the Stewart Fahs and Kinney study found in Appendix A of the text. Complete a critique of this study. Write no more than two or three sentences for each of the 17 content sections you identified in Activity 3. Make sure you have validated your list in Activity 3 with the appropriate list in the study guide answers.

1. _____

_____

_____

2. _____

3. _____

4. _____

5. _____

6. _____

7. _____

8. _____

9. _____

10. _____

_____

_____

11. _____

_____

_____

12. _____

_____

_____

13. _____

_____

_____

14. _____

_____

_____

15. _____

_____

_____

16. _____

_____

_____

17. _____

_____

_____

Check your answers with those in Appendix A, Chapter 19.

ACTIVITY 5

Some of you may have caught the research bug by now and are starting to wonder what it would be like to conduct a research study. Guiding you through the design and completion of a research study is beyond the scope of this text, but thinking through a few questions can be helpful. The first set of questions seeks information about general research activity in an agency. The second set addresses the availability of consultation for a research project.

If you are still thinking about a research project after you have collected the answers to the questions, consult a faculty member in your school of nursing. Most schools have a mechanism for independent study and many faculty would enjoy helping a student with such a project.

1. Choose a clinical problem that is of interest to you.

   _____

Research climate questions:

1. Is anyone studying some aspect of the clinical problem you identified?

   _____

2. Is there a research committee in the Department of Nursing? In the agency? Is it multi-disciplinary? Do they utilize nurse researchers?

   _____

   _____

   _____

   _____

3. What is the educational preparation of the senior nurse executive in your clinical setting? Of your supervisor? Of your head nurse? Of the senior nursing staff?

   _____

   _____

   _____

   _____

   _____

   _____

4. Are there any people in the setting who prominently advocate either conducting research or basing practice on research anywhere in the clinical agency or system? (This might be someone from another discipline.) Name them:

_____

_____

5. Summarize your answers to these questions. Come to a pro or con conclusion indicating whether you think this organization will facilitate or hinder research utilization if you attempt to solve a problem.

_____

_____

_____

_____

Availability of consultation questions: Continue to use your identified clinical problem as a way of focusing your questions.

1. Are there doctorally prepared nurses available for consultation either in your present clinical setting or at an affiliated university?

_____

2. If your answer to #1 is "no," are there master's prepared nurses available for consultation in your setting?

_____

3. If your answer to #2 is "no," are there doctorally prepared allied professionals in the setting who could be of assistance?

_____

4. List below the names and positions of all of the people you thought of when answering these questions.

_____

_____

_____

_____

5. Do nurses participate in nursing research? If they do, how are they involved? How are nurses involved in other types of investigative or research problems/projects?

_____

_____

_____

_____

_____

6. What facilities and services are available to you for pursuing research (library, computer searches, word processing, audiovisual department, etc.)?

_____

_____

_____

_____

_____

There are no specific answers for these questions. The questions are used to stimulate your attention to the need to utilize people and resources in the agencies where you are employed or are utilized as student placements.

Information concerning research in agencies can be obtained from the Office of Nursing Research, Staff Development, or Department of Nursing. Many units utilize committee structures to work together on problems or topics. Begin by asking your fellow colleagues, nurse manager, assistant head nurses, staff developers or unit clinical nurse specialists attached to your unit. Read the bulletin boards announcing agency activities or job placements. Many agencies will utilize newsletters or program announcements that can be found in nurses stations or placed in your pay envelopes. If you continue to have difficulty, ask your fellow nurses on the units. The increased communication between you and your colleagues can raise awareness about the level of research in the agency and the development of research projects.

POSTTEST

Using the suggested categories (content sections) and the format used in Activity 4, critique the Grey, Cameron, and Thurber study found in Appendix B of the text.

1. Introduction _____

   _____

   _____

2. Problem statement _____

   _____

   _____

3. Literature review _____

   _____

   _____

4. Theoretical framework _____

   _____

   _____

5. Definitions _____

   _____

   _____

6. Hypotheses/research questions _____

   _____

   _____

7. Methodology _____

   _____

   _____

8. Sample _____

_____

_____

9. Ethics _____

_____

_____

10. Instruments _____

_____

_____

11. Procedures - description of each specific step of the data collection process

_____

_____

_____

12. Results _____

_____

_____

13. Discussion _____

_____

_____

14. Interpretation of findings _____

_____

_____

15. Conclusions _____

_____

_____

16. Implications for nursing _____

_____

_____

17. Recommendations for future study _____

_____

_____

The answers to the posttest are in the Instructor's Resource Manual. Please check with your instructor for these answers.

REFERENCES

Grey, M., Cameron, M. E., and Thurber, F. W. (1991). Coping and adaptation in children with diabetes. *Nursing Research,* 40(3), 144-149.

Stewart Fahs, P. S. and Kinney, M. R. (1991). The abdomen, thigh, and arm as sites for subcutaneous sodium heparin injections. *Nursing Research,* 40(4), 204-207.

CHAPTER

20

Evaluating Qualitative Research

INTRODUCTION

Evaluating research with respect to the report's strengths, weaknesses, and applicability of the findings provides the critiquer with the essential tools in describing and explaining human phenomena.

LEARNING OBJECTIVES

On completion of this chapter, the student should be able to do the following:

- Identify the criteria for critiquing a qualitative research report.
- Describe the applicability of the findings of a qualitative research report.
- Construct a critique of a qualitative research report.

ACTIVITY 1

Qualitative research critiquing guidelines enable the critiquer to evaluate qualitative research reports.

1. Decide which of the following statements relevant to qualitative research critiquing criteria guidelines found in Table 20-1 of Chapter 20 in the text are correct and which are incorrect.

    a. Sampling procedures follow the random sampling criteria.
       Yes   No

    b. The researcher should describe the projected significance of the work to nursing.
       Yes   No

    c. The phenomenon of interest does not need to be clearly identified.
       Yes   No

    d. The subjects of the research do not need to be appropriate to the phenomenon being observed.
       Yes   No

e. The philosophical underpinnings of the research must be described in the research report.

Yes   No

f. The research report does not have to describe how the data were analyzed.

Yes   No

2. Several terms are unique to qualitative research. Match the definition in Column B with the appropriate term in Column A.

Column A   ·   Column B

1. _____ saturation β a. understanding researcher's thinking
2. _____ credibility ε b. sufficient sample size
3. _____ auditability A c. subject-behavior-environment specific
4. _____ fittingness D d. finding applicability
5. _____ context boundε e. personal experiences of subjects

Check your answers with those in Appendix A, Chapter 20.

ACTIVITY 2

1. The findings, conclusions, implications, and recommendations of qualitative research reports differ somewhat from the quantitative research reports. Complete the following statements regarding qualitative research reports.

a. The purpose of qualitative research is to _____ or

_____ a phenomenon or culture.

b. The goal of qualitative research is not to _____ or

_____ phenomenon.

c. The results of qualitative research are not _____ to larger groups.

d. The findings of qualitative research must be _____ for accuracy.

e. The critiquer of the qualitative research is responsible for determining whether the

findings accurately reflect _____ in another setting.

f. Findings from qualitative studies of culture must be viewed within a

_____.

g. Qualitative research should add to the existing body of knowledge and help to guide

_____   _____.

h. Qualitative research findings can lead to the development of

_____   _____ which are
useful to the nursing practice.

i. Qualitative research is grounded in the reality of _____

_____ with a _____

_____.

j. The findings of qualitative research provide the critiquer with direction on the focus for

_____   _____ related to the concept studied.

2. Using the Findings, Conclusions, Implication Recommendations Critiquing Guidelines
   for Qualitative Research found in Table 20-1 of Chapter 20, read the findings, discussion
   and recommendations, and further research sections of the article "Types and Meanings
   of Caring Behaviors Among Elderly Nursing Home Residents" by Hutchison and Bahr
   (1991) found in Appendix C of the text. For each of the 8 criteria, write a 2-3 sentence
   paragraph describing:

a. whether the criterion was met

_____

_____

_____

_____

_____

b. how the criterion was or was not met

_____

_____

_____

_____

_____

c. the research report's strengths and limitations based on each criterion

_____

_____

_____

_____

_____

3. After critiquing the findings, discussion and recommendations, and further research sections of Hutchison's and Bahr's article, explain:

a. how their research may affect your nursing practice

_____

_____

_____

_____

b. what further research ideas you can generate (other than those suggested in the article)

_____

_____

_____

_____

c. how you might replicate this study

_____

_____

_____

_____

Check your answers with those in Appendix A, Chapter 20.

POSTTEST

1. True   False   Qualitative research uses researcher interviews of subjects as one means of collecting data.

2. Validating whether research findings accurately reflect phenomenon in another setting is known as:

   a. credibility
   b. auditability
   c. fittingness
   d. confirmability

3. Being able to follow the qualitative researcher's line of thinking is known as:

   a. auditability
   b. credibility
   c. fittingness
   d. confirmability

4. When subjects in a qualitative research report recognize that what they are describing is their own experience, they are establishing:

   a. fittingness
   b. confirmability
   c. credibility
   d. auditability

5. True   False   Findings of qualitative research are generalizable to larger groups.

The answers to the posttest are in the Instructor's Resource Manual. Please check with your instructor for these answers.

REFERENCE

Hutchison, C. P. and Bahr, R. T. (1991). Types and meanings of caring behaviors among elderly nursing home residents. *Image: Journal of Nursing Scholarship,* 23(2), 85-88.

APPENDIX A

Answers to Activities

CHAPTER 1

ACTIVITY 1
1. c
2. b
3. d
4. a
5. e

ACTIVITY 2
1. D
2. B
3. C
4. D
5. A
6. B
7. A
8. C

ACTIVITY 3

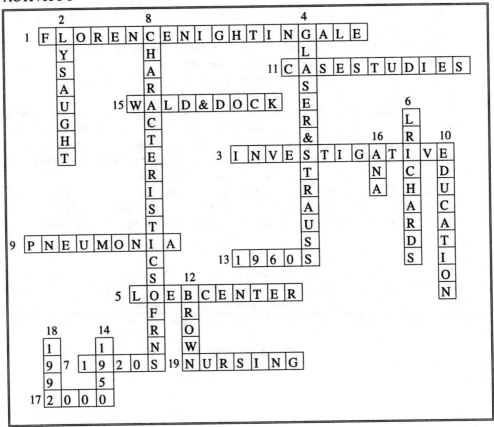

ACTIVITY 4

1. a. Stewart Fahs, RN, MSN
   Kinney, RN, DNSc
   b. Grey, PhD
   Cameron, MS, RN
   Thurber, PhD, RN
   c. Hutchison, RN, DNSc
   Bahr, RN, PhD

2. a. Appendix A - No
   Appendix B - Yes
   Appendix C - Yes
   b. Appendix A - Stewart Fahs, the first author, is a DSN candidate, and the second author, Kinney, has a doctorate in nursing science; therefore, between these two researchers there is sufficient educational experience to design and conduct the study. In addition, please note that this study was funded by an award from the National Center for Nursing Research, National Institutes of Health, which indicates that a panel of external reviewers examined the proposal and decided it had enough merit to fund its completion.
   Appendix B - Second author Cameron is a doctoral student who has progressed enough in her studies to achieve candidacy. Third author Thurber is doctorally prepared. Thus this team with two doctorally prepared nurses has the educational background to knowledgeably design and carry out this research study. Also, on reviewing the reference list it appears Grey has conducted prior research on this topic.
   Appendix C - Second author Bahr is doctorally prepared. Although in this study the first author was not doctorally prepared, in the biography section she thanks her dissertation committee composed of four doctorally prepared individuals, thus indicating a high degree of involvement of several doctorally prepared faculty.
   c. All of the authors in the three studies are affiliated with colleges or universities either as doctoral students or faculty. The academic titles range from lecturer to professor. Note: if no address is given for correspondence regarding the article, it is usually possible to reach the author through their university affiliation. Universities are listed in the U.S. post office zip code book by state, so addresses are easy to obtain.
   d. Appendix A: The Stewart Fahs and Kinney studied was funded by the National Center for Nursing Research. Appendix B: The Grey, Cameron, and Thurber study was funded by a grant from the University Research Foundation, University of Pennsylvania.

ACTIVITY 5

a. Continuing to conduct research on the topic of abuse in women
b. Developing theoretical perspectives
c. Conducting synthesis conferences into the area of abuse in women
d. Using nursing research studies to assist in legislative change

CHAPTER 2

ACTIVITY 1

1. S
2. U
3. U
4. S
5. S

6. U

ACTIVITY 2
1. g
2. h
3. e
4. d
5. a
6. c
7. f
8. b
9. j
10. i

ACTIVITY 3
Process 1: inductive
Process 2: deductive

ACTIVITY 4

Research Process	Nursing Process
1. Formulate and delimit the problem	1. Assessment
2. Review related literature	
3. Develop a theoretical framework	2. Planning
4. Identify the variables	
5. Formulate hypotheses	3. Implementation
6. Select a research design	
7. Collect the data	4. Evaluation
8. Analyze the data	
9. Interpret the results	
10. Communicate findings	

   c. The research process is quite similar to the nursing process. Eight of the 10 steps in the research process can readily be identified as being part of the nursing process.

   d. The major difference between the two processes is the number of steps, with the research process listing 10 and the nursing process only 4. However, the only two steps in the research process that are not readily apparent in the nursing process are Step 3 (develop a theoretical framework) and Step 10 (communicate findings).

CHAPTER 3

ACTIVITY 1
1. f
2. b
3. a
4. e
5. d

ACTIVITY 2
 1. tradition
    authority
    trial and error
 2. WICHEN (Western Interstate Commission for Higher Education) and was funded by
    United States Department of Health, Education and Welfare
 3. implications for practice
 4. use
 5. every
 6. no authority to make change
    no time to implement innovations
 7. Three of the following:
    start a journal club
    read research on my own
    start a research committee
    ask why I am doing this
    read "research briefs" in practice journals and professional organizational newspapers
    review CAI
    check to see if my agency has a downlink so I can attend conferences
 8. cost of health care is increasing
    containment of costs is a major issue
    quality of care is an issue for the consumer
 9. should not
10. bring about improvement in delivery of nursing care
11. Two of the following:
    Pew
    Kellogg
    Robert Wood Johnson
12. Two of the following:
    chronic illness
    self and community care
    the elderly

ACTIVITY 3
 1. The change in site would make it unnecessary to remove the patient to an area for total
    privacy in order to lift clothes to obtain an abdominal site for the injection. This could
    save time for the nurse. Rather, based on this study it could be given in an extremity when
    the situation warranted. The researchers also cited a source that indicated some patients
    were fearful about receiving an injection in the abdomen.
 2. a. Scientific merit -
       The researchers checked APTT on all subjects prior to the initiation of heparin therapy
       to make sure they were in the normal range and checked four hours after the first dose to
       see if the heparin had a different effect at any of the three different sites. Each site was
       checked for the occurrence of bruising at the site. The times for checking the research
       were established by previous research. The people who checked the sites had criteria
       for what to define as a bruise and had a high interrater reliability ($r = 0.94$ to 0.99).
       In addition, the size of the bruise was measured two ways. First, the widest diameter of
       the bruise was measured. Then a piece of plastic wrap was placed over the bruise and
       the bruise was outlined. The plastic was then traced onto a graph and the actual area

was calculated. The researchers even attempted to standardize the nurses' injection procedure by using videotape and a live presentation on the technique with training sessions held for new nurses.

b. Replicability -

The researchers were very specific on how the study and the statistical analysis were done, and any variances were explained. It would be very simple to take the information provided and develop a small or large study based on this research. The statistical design was strong and outcome variance was explained.

c. Relevance to practice -

The researchers spell out in the beginning of the study the practice relevance associated with this study. As they state, "use of the abdominal site for subcutaneous heparin injections may frighten the patient and inconvenience the nurse." (Stewart Fahs and Kinney, 1991, p. 204)

d. Importance as a client problem -

Stewart Fahs and Kinney (1991) report that Chamberlain (1980) noted the fear clients may experience with abdominal injections.

e. Feasibility for nurses to implement -

The study results would be very easy for nurses to implement. No advanced training, equipment, or change in techniques is required. The nurses can offer the patient a choice as part of his care. The only change that would have to be implemented would be to change the Policy and Procedure Manual's Standard of Care.

f. Risk-benefit ratio -

The patient is not in any danger or inconvenienced and is receiving the standard treatment. While this patient would not receive any direct benefit from the study, the information would benefit future patients.

3. Phase I: Validation

a. Scientific merit -

The researchers checked APTT on all subjects prior to the initiation of heparin therapy to make sure they were in the normal range and checked four hours after the first dose to see if the heparin had a different effect at any of the three different sites. Each site was checked for the occurrence of bruising at the site. The times for checking the site were established by previous research. The people who checked the sites had criteria for what to define as a bruise and had a high interrater reliability ($r = 0.94$ to 0.99). The size of the bruise was measured two ways. First, the widest diameter of the bruise was measured. Then a piece of plastic wrap was placed over the bruise and the bruise was outlined. The plastic was then traced onto a graph and the actual area was calculated. The researchers even attempted to standardize the nurses' injection procedure with videotape and a live presentation on the technique for all staff and training sessions held for new nurses.

b. Significance for practice -

The researchers spell out in the very beginning the practice relevance associated with this study. As they state, "use of the abdominal site for subcutaneous heparin injections may frighten the patient and inconvenience the nurse." (Stewart Fahs and Kinney, 1991, p. 204)

c. Strength of study -

Strong

Phase II: Comparative Evaluation

a. Substantiating evidence -

No similar study dealing with the site of injection is reported by the researchers.

b. Fitness of setting -
The factor that would inhibit utilization is the tradition of using only the abdominal site. The factors that facilitate utilization are no cost to implement change; no new training is necessary to implement change; and no risk to the patient is associated with the change. Rather, the patient could now be offered a choice of sites for the heparin injection.

c. Basis for practice -
Would require change of policy and procedure manuals to allow for change in site as a standard of practice.

d. Feasibility -
Excellent because of ease of change.

Phase III: Decision Making

a. Non-application must be the decision at this point in time. The change is not ready to be implemented because replication of this study is needed to support the findings.

CHAPTER 4

ACTIVITY 1
1. rational
2. dialogue
3. writer's point of view
4. a. preliminary understanding
   b. comprehensive understanding
   c. analysis understanding
   d. synthesis understanding
5. Three to four

ACTIVITY 2
1. b
2. b
3. a
4. b
5. a
6. a

ACTIVITY 3
1. a. Read abstract closely
   b. Skim complete article
   c. Highlight main steps of research process
   d. Write key variables at top of page
   e. Review old and new terms
2. a. Review unfamiliar terms
   b. Read additional sources
   c. Write cues, conceptual relations, etc., on copy of article
   d. State main idea in own terms
3. a. Be familiar with critiquing criteria
   b. Complete comprehensive reading
   c. Apply critiquing criteria to each step of the research
   d. Ask others to critique article, compare results

  e. Note on article how each part of the research measured up
 4. a. Review your own notes on the copy
    b. Summarize study in own words
    c. Complete one handwritten 5x8 card

ACTIVITY 4
Abstract 1
 1. depression, substance (chemical) dependence, social support, nurses
 2. quantitative (correlation study)
 3. Some possibilities: peer assistance participants, social support, "significantly related to," $(r = -.642, p < .001)$
 4. May know a chemically dependent nurse or student nurses. May be a psych/mental health nurse. May be a peer assistant.

Abstract 2
 1. Chest pain (reported and unreported), decision making, acute myocardial infarction, internal and external cues
 2. Qualitative (exploratory)
 3. Some possibilities: chest pain, purposeful sample, exploratory design, qualitative methods, decision making process
 4. May be coronary care nurse. May be med-surg nurse. May be interested in pain management or in client decision making.

CHAPTER 5

ACTIVITY 1
 1. Uncovers new knowledge that can lead to the development, validation or refinement of theories.
 2. Reveals appropriate research questions for the discipline.
 3. Provides the latest knowledge for education.
 4. Supplies practice with new knowledge especially as research-based nursing interventions.

ACTIVITY 2
 1. Clinical nurse - To implement research based nursing interventions; or to develop specific nursing protocols or policies for patient care based on several literature reviews; or to develop and substantiate specific QA, CQI, or TQM projects.
 2. Nursing faculty - To prepare lessons; or to develop and revise curricula; or to develop papers and presentations.
 3. Nursing student - To use as rationale for nursing interventions in nursing care plan; or to develop scholarly (research-based) papers; or to prepare oral presentations or case studies.

ACTIVITY 3
 1. B
 2. A
 3. B
 4. B
 5. A
 6. B

ACTIVITY 4

Choose from any of the following scholarly nursing journals for the five correct answers: *Advances in Nursing, AORN Journal, Applied Nursing Research, Archives of Psychiatric Nursing, Computers in Nursing, Heart & Lung, Holistic Nursing Practice, Image, Journal of Professional Nursing, Journal of Nursing Education, Journal of Nursing Scholarship, NA-COG, Nurse Educator, Nursing Diagnosis, Nursing & Health Care, Nursing Research, Nursing Science Quarterly, Research in Nursing & Health, Scholarly Inquiry for Nursing Practice, Western Journal of Nursing Research.*

ACTIVITY 5

1. a. Literature Review
   b. Review of the literature
   c. No title given. This is a typical introduction to a grounded theory study, because in this type of research the researcher will bring some knowledge of the literature to the study but does not usually do an exhaustive search of the literature. Instead, the researcher allows theory to emerge from the data, a process that will be described in-depth in Chapter 11. Also, please note the authors include the important disclaimer, "Throughout the review of literature, no studies or reports were found that comprehensively focused on ways residents are socially productive through caring acts, or what it means personally to a resident to engage in caring kinds of behaviors (p. 85)," indicating a major gap in information regarding this subject.

2. Yes
   It does read like a thorough detective story or a well-designed research proposal. The research first cited on the topic is in 1981, where angle of injection, aspiration and massage of tissue was studied. Then in 1984 three techniques for administering subcutaneous low-dose heparin on formation of bruises were studied. In 1988 a study compared two different techniques based on size of syringe and size of air bubble, change of needle and dry sponge technique; and in 1987 the variables of concentration and volume of heparin were studied. Two review articles were written on the topic in 1987 and 1988. Thus when this research was initiated in 1990 new variables to study were identified, which were the use of alterative sites and bruising.

ACTIVITY 6

1. S
2. P
3. S
4. S
5. P
6. P
7. P

CHAPTER 6

ACTIVITY 1

1. *Concept*: image or symbolic representation of an abstract idea
   Theoretical framework: provides a context for examining a problem
   Conceptual definition: conveys the general meaning of the concept, much like the definitions one would find in a dictionary

Operational definition: describes the procedures or operations that will be used to measure the concept as defined

2. a. concept
   b. conceptual definition
   c. conceptual definition
   d. theoretical framework
   e. operational definition

ACTIVITY 2

1. afterdrop, noninvasive measures of temperature, core temperature, severely hypothermic patient
2. uncertainty, hope, symptom severity, control preference, psychosocial adjustment, radiotherapy
3. cesarean birth information (the additional phrase "given in childbirth preparation classes" further explains the concept), maternal postpartum reaction to unplanned cesarean section
4. heart rate variability, anxiety, anger, denial, depression, acute myocardial infarction
5. body-image, self-concept, treatments (can be identified as a group or listed individually)

ACTIVITY 3

1. No
2. Yes
3. Yes
4. No
5. Yes

ACTIVITY 4

1. a. person or humans
   b. environment
   c. health
   d. nursing
2. a. B
   b. N
   c. B
   d. B
   e. N
   f. N
3. a. person (for item #2.b.)
   b. person or health (for item #2.e.); a case could be made for either concept
   c. person (for item #2.f.); yes, the focus is on nurses, which might have led you to think the concept of interest was "nursing," but the attention is being given to a characteristic of individual nurses and not to the practice of nursing

ACTIVITY 5

1. The Grey, Cameron, and Thurber study is the strongest simply because it has more sections evaluated as either "well done" or "OK."
2. The stronger a study is in technical areas the more likely one believes the results. As belief increases so does the probability that action related to that belief will occur and practice may be infuenced.

CRITIQUING GRID

	Well Done	OK	Needs Help	Not Applicable
1. If clearly identified - Could I find it?		F, G		H
2. Concepts				
a. conceptual definition(s) found		G	F	H
b. conceptual definition(s) clear		G		F, H
c. operational definition(s) found			F, G	H
d. operational definition(s) clear				F, G, H
3. Satisfied with operational definitions of conceptual definitions			F, G	H
4. Enough literature reviewed				
a. for an expert in the area				
b. for a nurse with some knowledge	G			
c. for a nurse reading outside of area of specialty or interest	F, H			
5. Thinking of researcher can be followed through theoretical material to hypotheses or questions	F, G			H
6. Relationships among propositions stated———clearly stated		F, G		H
7. Use of concepts is consistent from beginning to end	F, G	H		
8. Theory				
a. borrowed		F, G		H
b. findings related to nursing	F, H	G		
9. Findings related back to theoretical base, can find each concept from the theoretical section discussed in the "Results" section of the report		F, G		H

CHAPTER 7

ACTIVITY 1

1. e
2. b
3. d
4. a
5. c

ACTIVITY 2

1. It is a statement of purpose, not a problem statement.

    Criterion a. Yes - it does identify the variables paid work role and health risk.

    Criterion b. No - it does not clearly express the variables' relationship to each other.

    Criterion c. Yes - it identifies the population as older widows during their conjugal bereavement. It would be helpful to have an age-range specified for older widows.

    Criterion d. It could be rewritten to clearly point out the possibility of empirical testing. The author does this in the "Method" section by stating: "The following hypothesis was formulated: the independent variables of Work History and Work Attitude are statistically significant predictors of the dependent variable of Health During Bereavement, as measured by the Widowhood Questionnaire . . . ."

2. Criterion a. Yes - variables identified are thermal biofeedback combined with progressive muscle relaxation, progressive muscle relaxation alone, blood pressure.

    Criterion b. Yes - a reduction in blood pressure is predicted.

    Criterion c. No - a population is not mentioned.

    Criterion d. Yes - testability is implied.

3. Criterion a. Yes - variables identified are social support, depression.

    Criterion b. No - the variables' relationship to each other is not expressed.

    Criterion c. Yes - the population is chemically dependent subjects who were participants in a state legislated peer assistance program for nurses.

    Criterion d. No - the term used is explored, not measured; it would be clearer if the researcher proposed a relationship between an independent and dependent variable.

ACTIVITY 3

	Independent Variable	Dependent Variable
1.	CRTs	Birth defects
2.	Birth defects	Independence/dependence conflicts
3.	White wine	Serum cholesterol level
4.	Type of recording	Patient care
5.	Profession (MD or RN)	Extended-role concept of RNs

ACTIVITY 4

1. H_R; DH
2. H_R; DH
3. RQ
4. H_R; DH
5. H_R; NDH

ACTIVITY 5

1. RQ: Does the use of CRTs by pregnant women influence the incidence of birth defects?
   H$_O$: The use of CRTs by pregnant women has no effect on the incidence of birth defects.

2. DH: As is in the chapter
   NDH: There is a difference in the number of independence/dependence conflicts between individuals with and individuals without birth defects.

   H$_R$: As is
   RQ: Do individuals with birth defects have a higher incidence of independence/dependence conflicts than those without birth defects?
   H$_O$: There is no difference in incidence of independence/dependence conflicts between individuals with and without birth defects.

3. DH: There is a positive relationship between daily moderate consumption of white wine and serum cholesterol levels.
   NDH: Daily moderate consumption of white wine influences serum cholesterol levels.
   H$_R$: There is a relationship between daily moderate consumption of white wine and serum cholesterol levels.

   RQ: As is
   H$_O$: There is no relationship between daily moderate consumption of white wine and serum cholesterol levels.

4. DH: As is
   NDH: Patient care differs when recording methods (problem oriented vs. narrative) differ.
   H$_R$: As is
   RQ: Which method of recording (problem oriented or narrative) leads to more effective patient care?
   H$_O$: The recording method makes no difference in patient care.

5. DH: Nurses have a more positive view of the extended-role concept for nurses than do physicians.
   NDH: As is
   H$_R$: As is
   RQ: In what ways do nurses and physicians differ in the way they view the extended-role concept for nurses?
   H$_O$: There is no difference between nurses and physicians in their view of the extended-role concept for nurses.

CHAPTER 8

ACTIVITY 1

1. a. The setting for the study was not stated.
   b. The subjects were general medical and surgical patients.
   c. 101 subjects were in the final sample.
   d. The selection procedure was not described. Subjects with less than 25 mm of adipose tissue at the site and pretreatment APTT greater than 34 seconds were excluded. Four subjects were dropped for bruising, prior IV heparin, or being nonwhite. Subjects were randomly assigned to groups by use of a list of random numbers.
   e. There were 2 ways events were measured: laboratory blood coagulation tests and measurement of bruising diameter and surface area.
   f. Yes. The setting and subject selection procedure were not clearly specified, which could limit the ability to generalize the results to one's own practice or to replicate the study.

ACTIVITY 2
1. *Research design:* A blueprint for conducting a research study. It includes the procedures that will be used to control the entire research process. It identifies whether the study will be nonexperimental, quasi-experimental, or experimental.
2. *Accuracy:* Involves reviewing the entire study to make sure that all parts of it follow logically from the problem statement.
3. *Control:* The devices or methods used to keep the conditions of the study constant or the same during the time of the study.
4. *Feasibility:* Consideration whether the study is possible and practical to conduct, including cost, availability of subjects, time, expertise, and ethics.
5. *Homogeneous sampling:* A sample selected from the general population that is similar, especially in regard to extraneous variables involved in the study.
6. *Random sampling:* A process to ensure that every subject or item has an equal chance of being selected or assigned.
7. *Internal validity:* A term that indicates the degree to which a research study is internally consistent. It answers the question: "Can I believe that the results reported in this study were due to the causes that the researcher states?"
8. *External validity:* A term that indicates the degree to which the results of a particular study can be applied to the larger population of interest.

ACTIVITY 3
1. Maturation. The mother's confidence could be increased by any number of factors, including just caring for their infant over time. The time of measurement could be immediately prior to discharge. Use of a control group would strengthen the findings.
2. Instrumentation. The use of standardized calibrated equipment and training for the volunteers would increase the internal validity of the findings.
3. History. The increase in taxes could account for a decrease in the rate of cigarette smoking. Use of a control group and randomization would improve interpretation of the findings.
4. Selection bias. The differences in smoking cessation rates could be attributed to a number of motivational factors. Random assignment to groups is needed to strengthen this design.
5. Mortality. The program is not successful for single homeless women with preschool children. It is important to look at the make-up of the final study sample when the results are interpreted.
6. Testing. Taking the test repeatedly may lead to an increase in confidence and accuracy. Use of different outcome instruments and measures may be necessary.

ACTIVITY 4
Situation 1
Internal validity: ---X_____ -/+_____ +++
Rationale: There is not control. There is no way of knowing whether this teaching method would produce any different results than any other method. Because there was no measure of anxiety before the teaching experience, it is unknown if the teaching program reduced the client's anxiety.
External validity: ---X_____ -/+_____ +++
Rationale: The clients were used because of their convenience for the researcher. It is not possible to generalize to other populations because there is no way of knowing what relationship this group of clients has to the population of all preoperative clients.

Situation 2

Internal validity: ---   -/+   X+++

Rationale: The subjects were randomized to each experimental condition. The procedures were systematically completed on everyone with no indication that anything strange happened during the study.

External validity: ---   -/+   X+++

Rationale: Because the subjects were adolescent mothers and were randomly assigned to groups, the results are more believable and generalizable to the larger population of adolescent mothers. The study was conducted at only one large urban eastern U.S. teaching hospital and should be replicated in other settings.

ACTIVITY 5

An experimental design was appropriate to answer the research hypotheses. Although the sample was one of convenience, the researchers controlled some of the extraneous variables by using random assignment into groups; excluding nonwhites, persons with insufficient adipose tissue, and those with elevated coagulation times; and employing strict procedures for injection techniques, bruise measurement, and laboratory results. The study was feasible by using a convenience sample and staff nurses. The design flows logically from the literature review and the hypotheses. Generalizability may be limited by the sample selection and exclusion criteria. The results raise important questions regarding heparin injections and practice based on tradition rather than scientific evidence.

CHAPTER 9

ACTIVITY 1

1. a. Mother-infant pairs were randomly assigned into either the control or experimental group. Randomization is done to control for other variables which may impact the results of the study. That is, each group should be similar in makeup in terms of other factors which may affect the outcome, such as age, residence, or socio-economic factors.
   b. A control group received routine care and served as a comparison group to see if the extra intervention made a difference. No manipulation of variables (new intervention) was conducted with this group.
   c. The researchers manipulated the care received by the experimental group. The experimental treatment was the independent variable in this study.
2. Threats to internal validity are managed through randomization and use of a control group. Each group through random assignment is likely by chance to have the same experiences, history, maturation, or other factors, except for the intervention program being tested.
3. This study would have implications for practice if the intervention could be shown to be consistently effective. It is necessary to read the entire article and other related articles.
4. It would be difficult to interpret if the outcome was due to the intervention program or to some other factor, such as type of person assigned to each group.
5. It would be difficult to determine if the outcome of the study was any different from the outcome which occurred with routine care.

ACTIVITY 2

1.

	experimental group	pretest	experimental treatment	posttest
random assignment	control group	pretest		posttest
	control group		experimental treatment	posttest
	control group			posttest

2. You could use a table of random numbers generated by a computer to assign nurses to each group.
3. For a pretest for groups 1 and 2, you would administer a questionnaire to measure nurses' information and attitudes toward chemically dependent nurses. Groups 3 and 4 would not receive the questionnaire.
4. The experimental treatment is implementation of the teaching plan to provide information to groups 1 and 3. Groups 2 and 4 will not receive this teaching program.
5. The Solomon four-group design is particularly effective for studies in which pretesting alone may affect the outcome.
6. This type of design is particularly effective in ruling out threats to internal validity that the before-and-after groups may experience. It is effective for highly sensitive issues which might be affected by simply completing a questionnaire as a baseline pretest.

ACTIVITY 3

1. The researcher controlled for possible bias by randomly assigning patients to groups.
2. The after-only design is useful in situations where testing may affect the outcome or where it may be difficult or impractical to conduct pretests. The patients in this study were too ill to take knowledge and anxiety tests early in their recovery. The knowledge test may also have influenced the outcome. This design requires fewer subjects than the four-group design.

ACTIVITY 4

1. No. Since there was no random assignment in the beginning, it is impossible to predict that the two groups are equal and that the response is the result of the experimental intervention.
2. There are many possible explanations for this outcome. For example, the Thursday group members may have all come together on one bus from a facility that had a new dietitian managing their diets, helping them with weight loss and low salt diets, or there may be a nurse at the facility making sure that they take their medications regularly. The group could have increased their exercise level and lost weight as a result.
3. No. There was a lack of random assignment.

ACTIVITY 5

1. The researchers in this study would not be able to generalize their results to another group of patients because there was no initial randomization of groups. It is impossible to know if the groups were comparable at the beginning of the study.

2. I would not recommend a change to case management based on this study. I would need more studies with greater control over the research process to consider a change.

ACTIVITY 6

1. It is impossible to know what caused the drop in blood pressure. To gain this information, each person would have to be interviewed to determine what he or she was doing to cause a reduction in blood pressure.
2. It is definitely not possible to state a clear cause-effect relationship based on this study with one group.
3. A series of tightly designed and controlled experimental or quasi-experimental studies with well-defined variables should be conducted before it would be scientifically sound to change teaching content.

ACTIVITY 7

1. Music could possibly have an effect on blood pressure, but additional supporting studies are needed.
2. A comparison group with no music, or a comparison group with different types of music, would enhance interpretation of the findings.

ACTIVITY 8

Quasi-experimental designs are usually more practical, more feasible, and more adaptable to real-world practice.

CHAPTER 10

ACTIVITY 1

1. *Correlational*: Assesses the relationship between two or more variables.
2. *Cross-sectional*: Studies a problem within a given time frame. Provides variable control through design and sample selection.
3. *Ex post facto*: Studies a problem after the fact.
4. *Longitudinal*: Studies a question through time. Collects data from a group over time.
5. *Prediction*: Establishes a basis for using a variable (or set of variables) to predict perform-ance on another variable.
6. *Prospective*: Start in the present and move to the future. Similar to longitudinal studies.
7. *Retrospective* is the same as ex post facto.
8. *Survey*: Collects a lot of data usually across a wide field of interest. Frequently addresses several questions without going into great depth on any one question.
9. e
10. d
11. a
12. b
13. c
14. a
15. c
16. e
17. c
18. c

ACTIVITY 2

1. Correlational:
   Advantages: Increased flexibility when investigating complex relationships among variables; efficient and effective methods of collecting large amount of data; potential for practical application in clinical setting; foundation for future research; possible framework for investigating relationship between variables
   Disadvantages: variables beyond control; unable to manipulate variables; no randomization so cannot generalize findings; unable to determine causal relationship

2. Cross-sectional:
   Advantages: Collect data in shorter period of time; less threat to validity than when studied over time; takes broader perspective of population at given time; results more readily available in short time; less costly than longitudinal
   Disadvantages: Can't study variable over time; can't establish in-depth developmental assessment of interrelationship of phenomena; unable to determine if change that was predicted is related to change that occurred

3. Ex post facto:
   Advantages: Similar to correlational; offers higher level of control
   Disadvantages: Unable to draw causal linkage between two variables; possible alternative hypothesis reason for relationship

4. Longitudinal:
   Advantages: Each subject followed separately and serves as his/her own control; increased depth of responses can be obtained and early trends in data investigated; the researcher can assess changes in the variables of interest over time
   Disadvantages: Costly in terms of time, effort, and money; chance of confounding variables affecting interpretation of results; subjects may respond in socially accepted way to be congruent with researchers expectations; maturational changes occur

5. Prediction:
   Advantages: Used when one desires to forecast items such as how successful someone would be in an endeavor; often combined with retrospective design to obtain data; facilitates intelligent decision making with use of objective criteria
   Disadvantages: Requires sophisticated statistical techniques; does not imply a cause-and-effect relationship between chosen independent variables and dependent criterion variable; if predictor variables not chosen with sound rationale, study may not be valid

6. Prospective:
   Advantages: Like longitudinal; greater control than retrospective because degree of control can be imposed on extraneous variables
   Disadvantages: Often takes too long for evidence to become evident

7. Retrospective:
   Advantages and disadvantages similar to ex post facto

8. Survey:
   Advantages; large amount of information from large population; economic; surprisingly accurate
   Disadvantages: Information superficial, breadth not depth emphasized; requires expertise in sampling techniques, questionnaire construction, interviewing, and data analysis; time consuming and expensive if large scale

ACTIVITY 3

1. Type of design: cross-sectional; survey
   Advantages: Helped assess an important educational question; able to collect data from a

fairly large number of subjects

Disadvantages: Not generalizable; sample volunteers from one university; study would have had greater power if longitudinal; threats to internal validity with history changes

2. Type of design: descriptive survey; longitudinal

Advantages: Available population; noninvasive questionnaires used

Disadvantages: Reliability and validity of questionnaire not established; woman's perceptions of labor and delivery and postpartum may be altered by many variables; these were not studied

3. Type of design: descriptive; correlational; prospective

Advantages: Convenience sample that would not disappear from study; able to assess high risk factors in a population of women with high risk lifestyles

Disadvantages: Prospective study but women interviewed only during 3rd trimester; not generalizable; sample too small; non random but most of available population took part

4. Type of design: longitudinal descriptive

Advantages: Provided excellent photos of skin changes; provided self-perception of pain in relationship to nipple changes

Disadvantages: Only Caucasian women used; small sample size; identification of skin changes during pregnancy could provide baseline comparison; baseline data from non-nursing mothers should be collected for comparison; breastfeeding technique not con-trolled

5. Type of design: retrospective, descriptive

Advantages: Noninvasive; large sample can be found

Disadvantages: Only one area of country surveyed; small sample size limited to women seeking services of family-planning clinic

ACTIVITY 4

1. Survey: Send a questionnaire to a large number of women. This would allow for answers with least amount of threat.

2. Correlational: Could build on the survey above by identifying variables thought to be related to unwanted sexual experiences. Make sure the questionnaires addressed those variables.

3. Ex post facto: Identify groups of women who have had unwanted sexual experiences and those who have not. Interview (or give questionnaire to) each group.

4. Prediction: Request information on several variables believed to be related to unwanted sexual experiences. Based on these variables predict who would and would not have had the experience. Compare predictions with what the women have said.

5. Cross-sectional: The survey design would be cross-sectional if sent to all women at the same time.

6. Longitudinal: Identify a group of females and ask them about unwanted sexual experiences at specified intervals over a 10-year period of time.

7. Retrospective: Identify specific variable thought to be linked to unwanted sexual experiences and ask women who have experienced unwanted sexual experiences about these variables.

8. Prospective: Essentially the same as # 6

1. Any study could be unethical if anonymity not guaranteed. Study 6 (above) could be very intrusive, which could be considered unethical.

2. Most expensive would be Studies 6 or 8, followed by 3, 4, and 7. Studies 1, 2, and 5 are the least expensive.

3. Would not participate in Studies 6 or 8. Others would be OK.
4. Study 1 with some parts of 2.

ACTIVITY 5
1. Cross-sectional
2. Yes, needed to identify coping and adaptation to stress in different age groups of IDDM children
3. Yes
4. Yes
5. Yes
6. Yes
7. No, states further work needed
8. Possible explanation provided for finding that neither self-care behaviors or intercurrent stressors were predictive of adaptation
9. Concurrent validity assessments were made
10. No specific section on limitation; discussed need for longitudinal study of same set of subjects

CHAPTER 11

ACTIVITY 1
1. a. natural environments
   b. life context
   c. life context
   d. natural settings
   e. dynamic interaction
   f. context laden
2. a. B
   b. A
   c. B
   d. B
   e. A
   f. B
   g. A
   h. B
   i. A
   j. A
   k. B
   l. A
3. Quantitative Research:
   Identifies a Problem
   Reviews Related Literature
   Writes Research Hypothesis/Research Questions
   Selects Theoretical Framework
   Chooses Research Design
   Selects Methodology
   Collects Data
   Analyzes Data
   Communicates Findings

Qualitative Research:
Identifies a Phenomenon
Structures the Study
Gathers Data
Analyzes Data
Describes Findings
Generates Testable Hypothesis and/or Research Questions (when applicable)

ACTIVITY 2
1. a. True
   b. True
   c. False
   d. False
   e. False
   f. True
2. Senior citizen centers
   School age children
   Grade school children
   Neighborhoods
   Families
   Comparisons of humans from different ethnic, racial, and cultural groups
   Humans from different geographic regions of the country
3. Caring is an integral part of human behavior and human needs. We, as humans, need to give and receive care. Nursing is involved with giving caring. Yet through giving care, nurses also receive feelings of self-worth and actualization. This gives nurses purpose in doing and drives the profession of nursing.

ACTIVITY 3
1. a. D
   b. C
   c. B
   d. A
   e. A
   f. B
   g. C
   h. D
   i. D
   j. A
   k. B
   l. C
   m. D
   n. C
   o. D
   p. A
   q. B
   r. A
   s. C
   t. D
   u. C

      v. B
      w. B
  2. a. 4
     b. 2
     c. 3
     d. 1
     e. 2

ACTIVITY 4

  1. 1. f
    2. e
    3. d
    4. g
    5. c
    6. b
    7. a
    8. f
    9. b
   10. f

CHAPTER 12

ACTIVITY 1

1. Convenience sampling:
   Advantage: Easy for researcher to obtain subjects
   Disadvantage: Has greatest risk of bias because these samples can be self-selecting and not representative of underlying population
2. Quota sampling:
   Advantage: Assures that proportional representation of the sample occur
   Disadvantage: Contains unknown source of bias, or choice of variables for bias of stratification may be misleading
3. Purposive sampling:
   Advantage: Allows for selection of very specific sample elements
   Disadvantage: Researcher error or bias in selection leads to low external validity
4. Simple random sampling:
   Advantage: Guarantees that every element in the population has an equal chance of being in the sample
   Disadvantage: Is expensive in terms of time, money, and effort
5. Stratified random sampling:
   Advantage: Representativeness of sample enhanced
   Disadvantage: Is expensive in terms of time, money, and effort
6. Cluster sampling:
   Advantage: Is more economical than other probability sampling strategies
   Disadvantage: Has higher sampling errors than in simple or stratified random sampling, and very complex analysis is required
7. Systematic sampling:
   Advantage: Obtaining sample is more convenient and economical
   Disadvantage: It is possible to introduce bias through inadvertent loss of randomness

ACTIVITY 2
1. P
2. N
3. P
4. N
5. N
6. P
7. P

ACTIVITY 3
1. Quota sampling
2. Systematic sampling
3. Simple random sampling
4. Convenience sampling
5. Cluster sampling
6. Purposive sampling
7. Stratified random sampling

ACTIVITY 4
1. The sample consisted of white medical/surgical patients. Diagnoses, age, and gender were described. Subjects with bruising or previous IV heparin were excluded. The description is fairly complete, although the definition of white is not given. The sample appears to be one of convenience.
2. For this study the parameters are defined.
3. The study results, as noted by the researchers, are not generalizable to nonwhites. Also variation in ease of bruising was not controlled.
4. Criteria for eligibility are inferred from the description of the sample: white, medical/surgical patients, no IV heparin, no bruising at the site. In the procedure secion of the article, the authors state that persons with pretreatment APTT greater than 34 seconds were excluded, as well as persons with less than 25 millimeters of adipose tissue at the injection site.
5. See number 4
6. Yes
7. How the sample was selected is not stated. It appears to be a convenience sample. This method is appropriate in terms of feasibility and accessibility.
8. There could be selection bias if there was another factor affecting any of the variables at the time of the study.
9. 105 subjects seems appropriate for measurement of 3 different sites. No rationale were presented regarding sample size.
10. Informed consent was obtained as required by the Institutional Review Board.
11. The researcher appropriately discusses the limitations of generalizing beyond a white population and possible differences in bruising.
12. The authors recommend replication, additional variables to control, and additional areas to research to provide increased support for the findings.

CHAPTER 13

ACTIVITY 1

1. No, this is not an adequate explanation. The form should state both the risks and possible benefits and give the name, address, and phone number of the researcher.
2. No, this is not an adequate explanation. The researcher needs to describe in detail each risk that could occur as a result of participation in this study so that the patient is able to give an informed consent.
3. Yes, this is an adequate explanation of the anonymity and confidentiality section of an informed consent form.
4. I would share with the couple my concern that they were obviously interpreting the consent form very differently. I would urge them to call the researcher in for an explanation while they were both present. I would also offer to be present during the explanation. I would also urge them to write down all the questions they have for the researcher.
5. As a patient advocate, I would explain that they have the right to stop participation in the research at any time. I would also discontinue using the experimental procedure, as it appears to be causing harm to the patients.
6. I would state that confidentiality is one of the basic components of informed consent in the research process. I would urge him to meet with the institution's IRB to check on this matter.

ACTIVITY 2

1. Study A
   a. 1,2,4,5
   b. 3,6,7,8
   c. Minimum
   d. Yes
2. Study B
   a. 0
   b. 1,2,3,4,5,6,7,8
   c. Maximum
   d. No
3. Study C
   a. 4,5
   b. 1,2,3,6,7,8
   c. Maximum
   d. No

ACTIVITY 3

1. As specified by IRB
2. Ages 8-18 gave assent (all parents gave consent)
3. Verbal consent obtained on tape recorder

ACTIVITY 4

1. Respect for persons
2. Beneficence
3. Justice

ACTIVITY 5
Children, elderly, mentally ill, unborn, persons with AIDS, people in institutions, vulnerable populations, e.g., students or prisoners

CHAPTER 14

ACTIVITY 1
1. b
2. a
3. c
4. Researchers have a moral obligation and an ethical responsibility to protect the human subjects which may be participants in a study. Since the students are minors, the informed consent of their parents would be required prior to initiation of the research study. It is possible that data collected might have negative consequences (e.g., the students may be engaging in illegal behavior). Also, the researcher should have cleared the proposal for his study through the university's Institutional Review Board.

ACTIVITY 2
1. a, d
2. b, c
3. c
4. a

ACTIVITY 3
1. d
2. b, c
3. b, c, d
4. b, c, d
5. c, d
6. d
7. a, b
8. d
9. a, b
10. a, b, c
11. d
12. b, c, d
13. a, c
14. d
15. b, c, d

ACTIVITY 4
Exercise 1
Since the possibility of interpreting the strategies in differing ways exists, you may have some answers which differ from those provided. You may want to discuss these differences with your colleagues or teacher. Refer to Chapter 14 of the text for a more in-depth discussion of the answers.

1. a. questionnaire
    b. requires limited use of resources for implementation (time, money, ease in execution); anonymity of participants; limited researcher bias; can quickly discern subjects' knowledge
    c. may not be thoroughly completed; testing recently learned information may not be indicative of information retained over time; responses may reflect social desirability; test may not be a true measure of knowledge or the ability to apply knowledge in practice; test may not accurately reflect skill
2. a. interview
    b. can clarify questions; seek additional information; obtain personal information from subjects; high response rate
    c. time consuming; requires training for interviewer; subjects' responses may reflect social desirability; interviewer bias in the way questions are presented
3. a. questionnaire
    b. ease in administration; anonymity; easy to score responses; provides researcher with information that subjects may be uncomfortable in discussing
    c. may not be thoroughly completed; questions could be misinterpreted; responses may reflect social desirability; subjects may be uncertain of their feelings or feelings may change radically after they are home; may be unable to respond appropriately to those subjects that have an inadequate knowledge base
4. a. observation
    b. excellent way to study a specific variable of interest (nurse discussion of sexual activity with post-MI client); provides for depth of information that can be collected; use of videotape allows for repeated observations
    c. the problem of reactivity (subjects change behavior because they are being observed); bias of observer; training of the observer; may be time consuming and expensive; may be difficult to find different subjects to do pre- and post- observations, especially if there were a number of nurses participating in the inservice
5. a. observation
    b. excellent way to study a specific variable of interest; can provide extensive data; eliminates the problem of finding client subjects; observation can be viewed more than once
    c. the problem of reactivity; nurses role-playing may act differently than with clients; evaluation bias of the observer; training of the observer; time consuming
6. a. interview
    b. can clarify questions for clients; provides opportunity to collect rich data; enough time has lapsed for client/significant other to identify their concerns; good chance interview will collect desired information
    c. may be time consuming; may be difficult to directly evaluate the effectiveness of the inservice program for nurses; subject may be uncomfortable openly discussing the topic with the nurse; interviewer bias; client concern with social desirability
7. a. observation
    b. may be less intrusive than a videocamera; minimal cost involved; can be repeatedly listened to for evaluation; adequate way of capturing the dialogue of the interview; method could provide rich data
    c. reactivity may be a concern; the absense of non-verbal cues may limit the observers' ability to evaluate the interview; evaluation of the observation may be time consuming; it may be difficult to obtain subjects for pre- and post- inservice interviews; completing the observation soon after the inservice may not reflect actual retention of knowledge by the nurse

Exercise 2

1. nurses' skills in facilitating discussion with post-MI clients about their sexuality
2. inservice program
3. What effect does an inservice program have on nurses' skills in facilitating discussion of post-MI clients about their sexual activity?
4. Your answer to this question may differ based upon your ability to analyze the research study, to make relevant decisions about the type of data needed to be collected, and to think critically about the appropriateness of the various data collection methods. It is vital that you are able to support your choices with a clear rationale. Discussion of your ideas with colleagues may be a meaningful way to evaluate your choices and enhance your creative and critical thinking ability. Keep in mind the variable you are interested in measuring (the nurses' skills). Would it be best to measure immediately after the inservice or allow some time to pass? How much time? What type of information would you gather with a test? A role-play? A client interview? What affect might observation have on the data collection? Giving consideration to these questions will assist you in identifying the best method for data collection.

ACTIVITY 5

Case 1

1. physiological
2. This method of data collection provides for the exactness and accuracy required to measure differences in the effects of treatments.

Case 2

1. questionnaires
2. This strategy provides a data collecting method which enables the researcher to gather extensive information about caregivers' caring, conflict, and stress through the use of a number of instruments.

Case 3

1. existing data
2. This data collecting method allows the researcher to use data already in existence to answer a research question which was not considered when the data was originally created.

Case 4

1. interviews
2. This method of data collection allows the researcher to collect rich data that is of a highly personal and individual nature. Since a phenomenological study is concerned with subjects' perceptions, interviews provide a strategy for assuring that subjects can reveal their feelings, beliefs, and attitudes.

Case 5

1. observation and interviews
2. Interviews at their best can only provide information that the subject is consciouly aware of and willing to disclose. Observation provides the opportunity for the researcher to identify behaviors and actions which the subject may not be aware of or is unable to discuss.

CHAPTER 15

ACTIVITY 1

1. There is random error, or a threat to reliability. The researcher could do something to reduce test anxiety or use an alternate method of obtaining the information needed.
2. There is systematic error, reducing the validity of the study. The weights reported are not valid readings consistently.
3. There is a threat to reliability or random error. The research assistants should receive training and have a protocol to follow, and interrater reliability should be checked.

ACTIVITY 2

1. The scale could be developed based on literature, experience, or other means and then submitted to a panel of judges who are experts in the area. The items in the scale could be rated by the experts for the degree of agreement with the concept of maternal attachment.
2. To establish concurrent validity, the researcher could administer a second measure of confidence or a measure of a related concept, such as anxiety, at the same time as the new confidence measure. It would be desirable to have a high correlation between the results of the two measures. To establish predictive validity, there should be a high correlation between early and later measures of confidence and the outcome behavior.
3. For convergent validity, you would want to use another social support instrument to see if there was a strong correlation of the results from both instruments. For divergent validity, you could use an instrument to measure an opposing concept, such as loneliness, and expect to see a negative correlation between the results from the loneliness scale and the results from the social support instrument. That is, persons with high support are more likely to score low on loneliness.
4. The factor analysis should show items clustering around one of two different factors corresponding to the type of support. Ideally, each item should relate to only one of the factors.

ACTIVITY 3

1. Test-retest methods could be accomplished by giving the same test again at a later date and seeing if the two scores were highly correlated. Parallel or alternate forms, such as alternate versions of the same test, could also be used to establish stability.
2. Alternate forms would be better if the test taker is likely to remember and be influenced by the items or the answers from the first test.
3. a. Split half
   b. Cronbach's alpha
   c. Item-total correlation
   d. Kuder-Richardson (K-R 20)
4. Interrater

ACTIVITY 4

There is little information on the reliability of the APTT measures other than the blood was collected by laboratory personnel and a calibrated instrument and control batch were used to determine values. The use of APTT was appropriate to operationalize the concept of effective therapy in the first hypothesis. No discussion is given of strengths or weaknesses, or alternate forms of testing.

Interrater reliability of bruising measurement was conducted and was appropriate. Details of the method to establish reliability and the qualifications of the research assistants were not discussed. Pearson correlation coefficients ranged from r = 0.94 to 0.99, indicating high reliability. Concurrent validity was established with bruise surface area measures as the alternate method. The correlations between the two methods ranged from r = 0.86 to 0.91, again, a high degree of reliability. The developmental stage, previous use of the measures, or previous reliability or validity were not discussed.

Strengths and weaknesses of the buising measures were discussed. The surface area measurements were deemed more accurate and used in the data analysis. The researcher discussed use of a more precise computer scan of bruising as being more expensive, but more accurate.

Overall, the measures used in the study appear valid and reliable and the researchers provided the basic information needed to critique the study.

CHAPTER 16

ACTIVITY 1

1. 1. a
   2. a
   3. d
   4. b
   5. a or b
   6. b
   7. d
   8. a
   9. d
   10. b
   11. c
   12. d

2. a. Name of variable: Oxygen
      Level of measurement: Ratio
   b. Name of variable: States of sleep
      Level of measurement: Nominal
   c. Name of variable: Loneliness
      Level of measurement: Ordinal or interval
   d. Name of variable: Temperature
      Level of measurement: Interval (because it is being measured with a Fahrenheit scale; temperature can be measured on a ratio scale when the Kelvin scale is used [-237.15 degrees Kelvin = 0 degrees Celsius = 32 degrees Fahrenheit])
   e. Name of variable: Independence
      Level of measurement: Nominal or ordinal

3. a. Data are ordinal because the amount of pain being experienced at each time interval can be ranked. It was either more than or less than the pain experienced at other time intervals. Although it was possible to have a true zero (no pain present), it is impossible to assume that the amount of pain experienced when moving from 1 to 2 on the scale is the same amount of pain experienced when moving from 3 to 4.
   b. Nonparametric statistics would be the most appropriate to use.

ACTIVITY 2

1. a. CT
   b. V
   c. CT
   d. V
   e. CT
   f. CT
   g. CT

2. a. If one considers the use of the scale described as resulting in ordinal data, then the use of the median and the range would be indicated. If one considers this scale to be based on an interval level of measurement, then the mean and standard deviation would be used.
   b. The data are nominal, and the mode would be the usual measure of central tendency. Common practice would have the range as the measure of variation.
   c. Mean and standard deviation working with at least interval data.
   d. Mean and standard deviation because the data are ratio.
   e. Median and range; even though the variable (income) is at the ratio level of measurement, the distribution is skewed.

ACTIVITY 3

1. a 50.8
   b. Group: those who received information about the procedure only
      Variable: state anxiety scores
   c. Preinformation scores of the group who would receive information about the sensations associated with a barium enema (S.D. = 7.54)
   d. Yes. The calculation of the difference scores (d) agrees.
   e. "These results imply that sensation information enhances congruence between expected and experienced sensations while procedural information does not" (from the text of the study).

2. a. General medical (X = 65.2)
   b. S.D. = 20.5
   c. The General Medical Unit nurses' burnout scores varied more than burnout scores in the other groups.
   d. Even though the mean burnout score was the highest for the general medical unit nurses, the presence of the highest S.D. indicates that this group are more heterogeneous. May be an indication that the high mean score is the result of a few very high scores.
   e. You would want more information about their level of burnout. Is the high mean score the result of all nurses scoring higher, or did a few nurses have really high scores? Before planning any intervention, this information would be vital.

3. a. Clinic 1 would be the preferred clinic. The mean waiting time is longer, but the standard deviation is much smaller. Remember, 96% of the people who are waiting will be seen with ±2 standard deviations of the mean. The 96% in Clinic 1 will be seen in between 20 minutes and 60 minutes, while the 96% in Clinic 2 will be seen either immediately (no waiting time) or in up to 115 minutes. If you are a gambler and the chance of being seen immediately appeals to you, and if the difference between 60 and 115 minutes is not a bother, then you may choose Clinic 2, but those considerations override the statistically based decision.
   b. Mode
   c. B is the most variable and thus would have the biggest standard deviation.

CHAPTER 17

ACTIVITY 1

Set 1:		Set 2:		Set 3:	
1.	b	1.	b	1.	a
2.	a	2.	a	2.	b
3.	c	3.	a	3.	a
4.	d	4.	b	4.	a
				5.	b
				6.	b
				7.	b

ACTIVITY 2

1. There is no relationship between preoperative self-efficacy and postoperative ambulation, deep breathing, recall of expected events, and requests for pain medication.
2. There is no difference in reported sexual functioning between hypertensive and non-hypertensive clients.
3. There is no difference in the value placed on personal health between runners and nonrunners.

ACTIVITY 3

Hypothesis 2:
1. association
2. c
3. c
4. d

Hypothesis 3:
1. b. Dominant concerns expressed by four groups of children will be different.
2. b
3. c
4. e
5. a
6. independent
7. c or d

Hypothesis 4:
1. The hypothesis addressed differences and specifies a direction for those differences (i.e., towel bath clients will have lower postbath anxiety scores than conventional bath clients).
2. Anxiety scores are being measured. Depending on the orientation of the researcher, anxiety may be considered as measured on an ordinal scale or an interval scale.
3. There are two groups: towel bath and conventional bath.
4. Groups are independent. There is no reason to think that persons receiving a towel bath could influence the anxiety level of those receiving a conventional bath or vice versa.
5. Conclusion: If data are thought to be on an ordinal scale, then the Mann Whitney U could be used. If data are thought to be on an interval scale, then the independent t-test would be used.

ACTIVITY 4

Hypothesis 1:

1. ——
2. .05
3. .019
4. yes
5. rejected
6. supported or accepted
7. The results were statistically significant. The value of U obtained from the data in this study was greater than the value of U at the .05 level of probability. The null hypothesis that there was no difference between runners and nonrunners was rejected, which allowed for the support of the original research hypothesis.

Hypothesis 2:

1. There is no difference in anxiety scores between the two groups.
2. There is no explicitly stated preset level of probability. We can infer that the .05 was used and one tends to assume that the .05 is used if the preset value is not stated. Critiquers need to be wary and ask themselves or the researcher: Why wasn't the level of probability stated? In this particular case, the preset level was stated in a part of the study not quoted in this study guide.
3. .045
4. yes
5. rejected
6. support or accepted
7. There was a statistically significant difference in anxiety reduction between those clients who received a towel bath and those who received a conventional bath. These results would have occurred by chance only 4.5 times out of 100 replications of this study. The statistically significant results held only for the immediate postbath anxiety scores. One hour after the bath there was no difference in anxiety scores between those who received a towel bath and those who received a conventional bath.

CHAPTER 18

ACTIVITY 1

1. a. A
   b. B
   c. B
   d. B
   e. A
   f. A
   g. A
   h. B
   i. B
   j. B
2. a. Yes
   b. No
   c. No
   d. Yes
   e. No
   f. Yes

    g. No
    h. Yes
    i. Yes
    j. No

3. alternate sites to abdomen, thighs and arms
   assess patients' levels of fear and pain
   observe for and measure bruising
   use suggested measuring technique for bruising
   study various cultural groups receiving heparin therapy

4. procedure committee meeting
   speak with medical staff regarding policy/procedures for heparin administration
   ask staff to assess for levels of pain and fear in clients receiving heparin
   inform staff of research findings and suggest implementing new policy for heparin
      administration
   instruct staff on how to measure bruises
   devise log for staff to use in recording medical administration which alters injection
      sites

ACTIVITY 2

1. a. Yes
   b. No
   c. Yes
   d. Yes
   e. Yes
   f. d
   g. c
   h. a
   i. b
   j. c

2. Suggested new title: "Differences in Surface Area Bruising Among Sites 8, 60, and 72
   Hours Postinjection"

3. different title
   add sample size
   correct p value error
   add "all three sites" to injection category

ACTIVITY 3

1. age and physical maturity impact adaptation to diabetes in children
   preadolescent and adolescent patients differ significantly in psychological, social, and
      physiologic adaptation to diabetes
   anxiety and depression are more common in adolescent diabetic patients
   metabolic control of diabetes and psychosocial adjustment worsen with increasing age
   adaptation may be a developmental problem rather than due to illness
   management approaches to diabetes must be age appropriate
   preadolescents and adolescents differ significantly in the manner in which they cope
      with illness
   adolescents with diabetes use more avoidance coping behaviors resulting in poorer
      adaptation and metabolic control

2. The study does not use a comparison group. Only subjects with diabetes are used so the investigators cannot be sure if adaptation is a developmental problem or one due to the illness.

   The study was conducted over a short period of time. A longitudinal study of children from preadolescence through adolescence may have had different results.

   The subscale of the A-Cope tool may be a weak measure of social support.

   Other tools in the article had spurious results.

   The subjects were asked to complete several instruments. Did this overwhelm the subjects, thus clouding the findings?

3. avoidance of the problem

   seek out friends for support

   fail to follow insulin regimen

   anger, depression

   may do fine now, but that could change as he grows older

4. support group for child and parents

   patient teaching on adolescent diabetes

   arrange home health visits or follow-up visits for the family to see how they are doing

   social services may help to identify need for counseling or therapy for patient and family

ACTIVITY 4

1. Performing admission and ongoing assessments of nursing home residents can assist in evaluating their potential and/or actual socially productive manner.

   Viewing nursing home residents as both givers and receivers of care who are capable of benefitting others through their caring is essential in nursing care of the elderly.

   Nursing must realize that for nursing home residents, being caring of others is important to them and helps them keep from focusing on their personal limitations and problems.

   Nurses must realize that caring affects nursing home residents' sense of personal identity. It may help to reduce their mental and physical deterioration.

2. Ask residents to write letters for other residents who cannot write.

   Ask residents to help other residents organize their belongings in their rooms.

   Ask residents to cut up the food on other residents' trays for those unable to do so.

   Ask residents to brush the hair of another resident unable to do so.

   Note: Nursing Home Policies and Procedures will dictate the limits of nursing home residents' activities in helping other residents.

CHAPTER 19

ACTIVITY 1

1. _*_ a.
   _*_ b.
   ___ c.
   _*_ d.
   ___ e.
   ___ f.
   ___ g.
   _*_ h.

In this activity a, b, d, and h are specifically research-focused. They have been created and published for many different topics and research interests.

The *Journal of Obstetric, Gynecologic, and Neonatal Nursing* is written by the AWWON association that focuses on nursing practice issues in that field. The publication does have a few nursing research articles as they relate to practice problems or questions.

The remaining three publications, *Nursing 93*, *American Journal of Nursing*, and *RN*, are written specifically for staff nurses in clinical agencies dealing with varied clinical focus problems, issues, and concerns. These three publications do not focus a major portion on nursing research topics.

3. a. introduction
   b. methodology
   c. results
   d. discussion

ACTIVITY 2

1. b
2. a
3. b
4. c
5. a
6. c

ACTIVITY 3

1. Introduction
2. Problem statement
3. Literature review
4. Theoretical framework
5. Definitions
6. Hypotheses/research questions
7. Methodology
8. Sample
9. Ethics
10. Instruments
11. Procedure
12. Results
13. Discussion
14. Interpretation of findings
15. Conclusions
16. Implications for nursing
17. Recommendations for future study

ACTIVITY 4

1. Introduction:
   Page 204. The authors were concerned that many hospitalized medical patients are frightened to use the abdominal site for subcutaneous heparin injection even though it has been suggested that this is the site of choice. Paragraph in italics above the body of the article is the beginning introduction.
2. Problem statement:
   Page 204. ". . . study was undertaken to determine whether alternate sites were effective in accomplishing the goals of low-dose heparin therapy and to identify any differences in bruising at the injection site."
3. Literature review:
   Page 204. Discussion of various studies and other articles providing information concerning this issue.
4. Theoretical framework:
   There is no specific discussion of a conceptual or theoretical framework. The research study is based on the need for low-dose thrombophlebitis.

5. Definitions:
   There are no specific lists of definitions of terms in the article. The authors assume you understand the concepts, terms, and key words without specifying their definitions.

6. Hypotheses/research questions:
   The three hypotheses are listed on pages 204-205. These hypotheses were appropriate for the study and could be answered by the completion of the research study.

7. Methodology:
   The study involved a quasi-experimental study involving repeated measures of administering three injections of sodium heparin in three sites: abdomen, thigh, and arm.

8. Sample:
   The initial sample consisted of 105 subjects, while the final sample consisted of 101 subjects classified as medical/surgical patients. All of the subjects were white since there was no interrater reliability for measuring the bruise measurements on dark-skinned individuals. Page 205 lists other demographic data of the sample.

9. Ethics:
   The authors did not discuss any of the ethical issues, nor do we know if they obtained informed consent to perform the study. However, the study was supported by the National Center for Nursing Research, National Institutes of Health. The approval of the Center for Nursing Research involves full client and agency informed consent. I believe the authors' not mentioning the consent was more of a matter of oversight than failure to obtain consent for research.

10. Instruments:
    The research study did not involve survey research; therefore, there is no discussion of data collection instruments. However, there had to have been documentation sheets for demographic data and recording the calculations of the bruises as well as recording the subjects receiving the sodium heparin.

11. Procedures - description of each specific step of the data collection process:
    Pages 205-206 itemize the specific procedures used for the study and the administration of the sodium heparin.

12. Results:
    Page 206 lists the results of the study by two categories: bruising and size of the bruises.

13. Discussion:
    Pages 206-207 indicate the discussion of the study. The discussion section also includes the authors' interpretations of the findings, implications for nursing, and the recommendations for future study.

14. Interpretation of findings:
    There is no separate section for interpretation of findings, but rather it is placed within the results and discussion section.

15. Conclusions:
    There is no separate conclusions section; it is placed within the discussion section.

16. Implications for nursing:
    The results of this research study demonstrated that sodium heparin could be given safely with the same type of bruising at all three sites (abdomen, thigh, arm). The nursing community assumed that the only safe place to give sodium heparin was in the abdomen. The study demonstrated no difference of bruising among the three sites.

17. Recommendations for future study:
    The recommendations for further study section is placed in the discussion section and not in its own section. In further research the time between measuring bruise after administra-

tion of medication should be lengthened. The authors believe the study should be repeated to allow each subject to be their own control and there should be research involving non-white subjects. The study did not identify the subjects' perceptions of their bruises nor whether there were any physiologic or psychologic reactions to their own bruises. The authors believed that these points would be strengthened in further research.

CHAPTER 20

ACTIVITY 1
1. a. No
   b. Yes
   c. No
   d. No
   e. Yes
   f. No
2. 1. c
   2. a
   3. e
   4. d
   5. b

ACTIVITY 2
1. a. describe, explain
   b. predict, control
   c. generalizable
   d. validated
   e. phenomenon
   f. context
   g. nursing practice
   h. research instruments
   i. human experience, particular phenomenon
   j. further research
2. The Hutchison and Bahr study is well done. Each of the criteria was met and met in a very readable style. It was easy to follow the thinking of the researchers and to follow the study from its beginning to its end. The setting of the study provided the only real limitation, but the need for such a setting was understandable.
   The purpose of asking you to think through each of the criteria is to provide you with practice in judging a study for yourself. You may or may not agree with the conclusions of others. You need to know, however, why you agree or disagree, so take the time to think through each item. Talk over your conclusions with a peer or with the instructor.
3. Once again the intent is for you to think through the implications of this piece of research for your practice. How will it help you be a better nurse? What other clinically based questions come to mind as you think about this study? As you think about replicating this study, review the identified limitations. How would you modify the study to address identified limitations?

Appendix B

Self-Care Actions of Healthy Middle-Aged Women To Promote Well-Being

Donna L. Hartweg

The purpose of this study was to describe self-care actions that healthy middle-aged women perform to promote well-being. The heterogenous sample of black and white women (N = 153) ranged in age from 40 to 59. Subjects responded to a structured interview guide based on Orem's Theory of Self-Care and a developmental change list. Women identified 8,693 diverse self-care actions that promote well-being. Using content analysis, actions were categorized by the purpose for which the action was performed. The majority were related to universal self-care requisites, with self-care actions related to categories of activity and social interaction most frequently cited. One fourth were self-care actions related to developmental changes experienced in middle age. Many self-care actions were performed to meet multiple purposes or requisites. When demographic variables were correlated with self-care actions, education, age, and number of children were significantly correlated with types of self-care actions.

Nursing research has historically focused on self-care actions related to the physical/functional health of individuals, with limited efforts to understand practices that promote well-being. Recent studies have emphasized the importance of well-being as a component of being healthy in women (Woods et al., 1988) and the need to advance this more positive construct of health (Kulbok & Baldwin, 1992).

The purpose of this study was to describe the specific self-care actions that healthy middle-aged women perform to promote well-being and the relationship of these actions to age, sociocultural orientation, family systems factors, and work patterns. Well-being was defined as a person's subjective or "perceived condition of existence," or, more specifically, as experiences of contentment, pleasure, and happiness, spiritual experiences, and movement toward one's ideal and achievement of human potential (Orem, 1991). Well-being, viewed as different from physical health, was also defined as structural/functional integrity (Orem, 1991). Both definitions are similar to outcomes of health-promotion and health-protection actions identified by Pender (1987). The former refers to practices that increase well-being; the latter to practices related to avoidance, treatment, or recovery from disease.

Review of Literature

Few studies have explored health practices or self-care actions performed to promote well-being in any population, although analyses of findings from related studies have generated action categories related to well-being as positive thinking, use of mind (Laffrey & Crabtree, 1988), psychological, mental, or emotional well-being (Harris & Guten, 1979), personal or emotional health (Hautmann & Harrison, 1982), and cognitive-affective types (Prohaska, Leventhal, Leventhal, & Keller, 1985). Kolanowski and Gunter (1985) reported the only study in which the focus was to identify self-practices or approaches to health that contributed to well-being. Although the study was limited to 26 healthy, retired career women, the findings demon-

Reprinted with permission from *Nursing Research*, 1993, Vol. 42, No. 4, pp. 221-227. Copyright 1993, American Journal of Nursing Company.

strated the ease with which women recalled and identified actions that promote well-being. The two most frequently identified action types were those related to communicating with others (social connectedness) and physical activity.

Freer (1980) conducted an exploratory study on self-care practices of 26 women, ages 35 to 44. Although the focus of the study was on medically oriented illness practices, the women identified 634 actions that made them feel better, 53% of which were related to social interactions. Although the sample was exclusively white and drawn from those attending a medical clinic, the ability to identify specific self-care practices that promote well-being was relevant to the present study.

By definition, health promotion has ties to self-care that promote well-being. Walker, Volkan, Sechrist, and Pender (1988) compared the health-promoting lifestyles of young and middle-aged adults (ages 35-54) to those of older adults. Using the Health-Promotion Lifestyle Profile (HPLP) (Walker, Sechrist, & Pender, 1987) to describe those practices that promote well-being and self-actualization, the investigators found that women of all age groups engaged in more actions related to the following dimensions than men: health responsibility, exercise, nutrition, and interpersonal support. Although the HPLP has been tested extensively, studies have suggested that the forced-choice nature of the instrument limits the diversity of responses in ethnic and culturally diverse groups (Davidson, 1988; Foster, 1987; Riffle, Yoho, & Sams, 1989), supporting the use of an open-ended approach when investigating actions related to well-being.

Orem's (1991) general theory of nursing has been used extensively as a framework for self-care research, although primarily with populations with specific diseases. In one of the rare studies on healthy population, Woods (1985) classified universal self-care activities and patterns of illness or symptom-related self-care of young adult married women, ages 20-40. Findings supported the frequency of self-care, with the majority of responses re-

lated to illness-oriented self-care, such as sympton prevention. Few nonmedical self-care practices, such as nutrition and exercise, were identified. Woods proposed that the open-ended data collection procedure and the Western emphasis on medication contributed to the limited number of nonmedical self-care practices. Although Woods did not distinguish self-care to promote well-being from self-care to promote health, the methodological issues raised supported the need to develop specific, comprehensive self-care questions in exploratory studies.

Investigators (Dan & Bernhard, 1989; McElmurry & Huddleston, 1991) emphasized the need to describe self-care knowledge and actions of middle-aged women, particularly as they relate to changes and symptoms experienced during middle age. When research and lay literature on physical, social, and psychological changes and needs of middle-aged women were reviewed, no studies identified specific actions related to these developmentally specific needs. However, selected coping strategies were identified for such distinct changes as hot flashes (Germaine, 1984; Stevenson & Delprato, 1983; Voda, 1981) and vaginal dryness (Dan & Bernhard, 1989; Leiblum, Bachmann, Kemmann, Colburn, & Swartzman, 1983). The focus of the literature was limited to symptoms of middle age. Self-care actions directed to more positive aspects of middle age, such as those described by Neugarten (1968), have not been reported. This supported the need for a comprehensive approach to investigation of developmental changes of middle age.

Orem's (1991) self-care requisites, or purposes for which individuals perform self-care, were selected as the organizing framework and are of three types: (a) universal self-care requisites are "common to all human beings during all stages of the life cycle, adjusted to age, developmental state, and environmental and other factors"; (b) developmental self-care requisites are "associated with human developmental processes and with conditions and events occurring during various stages of the life cycle (e.g., prematurity, pregnancy) and events that can adversely affect development"; and (c) health-deviation self-care requisites are "associated with genetic and constitutional defects and human structural and functional deviations and with their effects and with medical diagnostic and treatment measures" (Orem, 1991, p. 125).

Method

Sample: One hundred fifty-three healthy women, ages 40 to 59, comprised the sample. To achieve diversity in race, socioeconomic status, family, and work patterns, women were recruited through multiple methods, including the use of contact persons in minority businesses and housing projects and the distribution of flyers to targeted groups.

Interviews were conducted with 58 black and 95 white women whose median age was 49 years. Educational level ranged from those completing eighth grade to those with graduate school preparation, with the majority (67.4%) having some college education. Total annual household income ranged from $700 to $400,000, with a median of $35,000. Over 35% were below the 1988 federally determined median incomes for black and white Americans. The majority (64.7%) were married or in a sustaining relationship. The mean number of children was 2.9, with a range of zero to 12. Over 55% of the women worked full-time for wages, 15% worked part-time, and 25% were not employed outside the home.

Questionnaire: Self-care actions related to universal, developmental, and health-deviation self-care requisites (Orem, 1991) were recorded on a theoretically derived structured interview guide and developmental change list form. Actions performed to meet requisites that were unclassifiable as a universal, developmental, or health-deviation self-care requisite were labeled as "emerging" for subsequent latent content analysis (Holsti, 1969).

Self-care actions to meet universal requisites of food/water, activity, rest, solitude, social interaction, elimination, air, hazards, and normalcy (self-esteem/self-image) were generated from questions developed from

Orem's general sets of actions related to self-care, resulting in creation of subcategories of universal requisites. For example, the category of activity contained four types of activity: physical activity, interests/talent activity, spiritual activity, and intellectual activity. The following question prompted responses to the need for spiritual activity: "Are there any spiritual/religious activities you do which help your sense of well-being?"

Responses to specific developmental requisites of middle age were generated through a change list of 110 physical, psychological, and social changes/events that have been related to middle age. The comprehensive list was developed from a thorough review of both scientifc and lay literature. Examples of changes include the following: (a) physical changes, such as hot flashes, reading (vision) problems, weight gain, vaginal dryness, and change in menstrual pattern; (b) psychological changes, such as increased sense of freedom, increased sense of resourcefulness, change in sense of time, feelings of depression, and awareness of mortality; and (c) social changes, such as children leaving home, children returning home, death of parent, change in spending ability, and change in satisfaction in personal relationships. Self-care actions related to the six health-deviation requisites were also solicited; for example, going to health clinics to see doctors or nurses for routine care.

The following open-ended question was presented first to prompt identification of actions unrelated to Orem's model: "Would you tell me about the self-care actions, or those things you do, for your well-being?" The women were then asked to identify the purpose for engaging in the action.

Consensual validity of the interview guide with Orem's (1991) model was established with experts on Orem's theory; content validity of the change list with four experts on midlife changes in women; and face validity with women representative of the sample. A pilot study was conducted with 10 women from various educational levels and backgrounds. Interrater reliability on the self-care

Table 1. Summary of Self-Care Actions to Meet Universal Self-Care Requisites

Classified Action Type	f	% of Universals	% of Total	Range Min.	Range Max.	M	SD
Food	789	13.4	9.1	0	16	5.2	3.5
Activity	1314	22.4	15.1	2	21	8.9	3.9
Rest	495	8.4	5.7	0	11	3.2	2.0
Solitude	358	6.1	4.1	0	11	2.3	1.9
Social interaction	1079	18.4	12.4	1	16	7.1	3.0
Elimination	437	7.4	4.8	0	8	2.9	1.7
Air	226	3.9	2.6	0	6	1.5	1.3
Hazards	548	9.4	6.3	0	12	3.6	2.1
Normalcy	621	10.6	7.1	0	11	4.1	2.2

Note. $N = 153$; total $f = 5867$.

actions among three interviewers and intrarater coding reliability by the principal investigator were 81% and 91%, respectively, acceptable levels for exploratory research (Miles & Huberman, 1984).

Procedure: The interviews were completed in the setting of the woman's choice, such as home, work setting, or community agency. After signing a consent form and completing the demographic questionnaire, the women were introduced to the concept of well-being. Examples were presented to distinguish self-care directed toward physical/functional health from self-care to promote well-being. Examples were selected carefully to decrease the tendency to provide socially desirable responses. All interviews followed an identical format. The primary investigator reviewed tapes periodically to ensure consistency in approach.

Following identification of self-care actions and related purposes, the women were asked to review the list of self-care actions and state the effectiveness of each action in promoting well-being. A scale of 0 to 100 was used, with 0 as no effectiveness and 100 as maximal effectiveness. This review provided validation of self-care as an action to promote well-being or physical/functional health. The taped interviews ranged in length from about 50 minutes to nearly 3 hours, with an average of 90 minutes.

All responses were coded by the investigator using decision rules validated by experts on Orem's theory. Actions were coded according to the purpose for the action. A response such as, "I walk four miles a day to socialize with my neighbors," was classified as a self-care action to meet the requisite of social interaction, not physical activity. Self-care actions that could not be classified as meeting known universal, developmental, or health-deviation self-care requisites were classified as "emerging," designating a requisite unaccounted for in Orem's general theory of nursing.

Results

Self-care actions were analyzed by manifest content analysis (Holsti, 1969), and the resultant datasets were analyzed using bivariate correlations and multivariate statistics. The 153 healthy women deliberately performed 8,693 diverse self-care actions to promote well-being. These were normally distributed in the sample and ranged from 14 to 117 per woman ($M = 56.8$, $SD = 19.5$). Over 67% of the actions were performed to meet the universal requisites, with one fourth (24.4%) performed for a developmental purpose. Fewer than 8% (7.6%) were performed to meet the health-deviation requisites. Approximately

4% could not be classified.

Universal: The women identified 5,867 self-care actions related to the universals. The range was 9 to 77 ($M = 38.3$, $SD = 12.7$). (See Table 1.) In the two universal categories with highest frequencies, the average number of "activity" actions was 8.9 ($SD = 3.9$), and the number of "social interaction" actions was 7.1 ($SD = 3.0$). The subcategory of hazards had the highest frequency of total actions related to universals (9.4%) and accounted for the highest percentage of all self-care actions (6.3%). Examples from each of the universal categories are presented to describe the diversity of self-care actions that women identified as promoting well-being.

Food/Beverages: Self-care actions that promote well-being included the deliberate avoidance of foods/beverages such as alcohol, caffeinated drinks, and chocolate. A habit that promoted well-being was eating at the table and not in front of the television. In response to a questions on actions to enhance the pleasurable experience of food, one woman cited "coming to the soup kitchen," suggesting that environment was a factor in promoting well-being through intake of food.

Activity: Women performed diverse activities related to the four activity subcategories. Walking was a frequently identified physical activity performed by women to promote well-being. Other individual responses included the following: "I hang wash on the line" and "I dance every day to all kinds of music around the house." Activities related to talents and interests exemplified the diversity in women's lives: "I sing in the church choir for fun," "I read," and "I like to take care of my plants—they're little trophies." Examples of religious and spiritual activities performed to promote well-being varied from those related to organized religious activities to spiritual activities related to nature: "Travel to see aspects of nature, such as the Redwoods—for spiritual reasons." Reading and going to work were commonly cited intellectual activities.

Rest: Common activities in preparation for sleep included reading, watching television, rocking, physical preparation such as bathing and showering, and mental preparation. Other activities included the selection of special drinks and complex rituals. Many of the activities used in preparation for sleep were also used as techniques for general relaxation, such as "take long bath, use scented candles, turn out lights."

Solitude: Women identified activities, such as "I walk to be alone and think," and "I read novels for diversion—to get away." To promote freedom, a category within solitude, women said, "Saving money gives me a sense of freedom" and "spending money...that's freedom."

Social Interaction: Common actions that promoted well-being included writing letters, sending cards, telephoning friends and relatives, and walking with friends and significant others. Making financial and time sacrifices for other people were common actions performed to promote well-being Diverse actions, such as volunteer work, were deliberately performed to help others.

Elimination: Many women identified increased water intake as an action to meet the elimination self-care requisite. Women responded to personal hygiene questions by citing many of the same actions that were used as examples in the question, such as brushing teeth, showering, and special care after menstrual periods. Many black women described douching after menstruation as a common practice.

Air: A general question elicited many responses related to avoiding smoke and providing for clean, fresh air in the home. Actions to enhance the pleasurable experience of breathing were diverse, such as "I breathe potpourri mixtures in stores" and "I'm taking classes on growing herbs and making potpourri."

Hazards: Common actions included those that were cited in the question, such as locking doors and wearing seatbelts. However, many were deliberate behaviors of women to keep themselves feeling safe: "I wear hats for body safety—to prevent losing body heat—it's not fair to my body" and "I teach kids about not smoking/taking drugs—helps me feel safer."

Table 2. Frequencies and Percentages of Self-Care Actions to Meet Health-Deviation Self-Care Requisites

Classified Action Health-Deviation Type	f	% of Type	% of Total
Routine care	304	45.8	3.5
Symptom care	153	23.0	1.8
Diagnostic, e.g., mammograms	146	22.0	1.7
Care for side effects	2	.3	.0
Adjusting feelings	5	.8	.1
Adjusting lifestyle	41	6.1	.5
Other	13	2.0	.1

Note. $N = 153$; total $f = 664$.

Another woman exemplified the interaction of rest and prevention of hazards: "I'm sure windows are locked and sleep in the front room on the couch so that I can see the entrance from the couch—I won't sleep in a closed room."

Normalcy: Many of the women's responses were mental actions, those eliciting pride from accomplishments. Actions that women identified as related to self-image included care of hair, nails, skin, and selection and care of clothing. Weight control actions that enhanced well-being were also stated, such as, "I swim a quarter of a mile (40 minutes) two times per week, so I won't look like a fat pig." Actions related to self-concept included "I play mental games. At singles' dances, I believe I'm the best thing walking through the door."

Developmental: The women identified 2,126 self-care actions deliberately performed to meet developmental requisites. Over 94% of those were performed in response to the 110 specific physical, psychological, and social changes/events associated with middle age. The average number of actions was 13.1 ($SD = 8.8$), with a range of 0 to 49. To focus on developmentally specific actions that affect well-being, women were asked to identify the self-care action related to the change only if the change had occurred since turning 40 and if it affected well-being. Examples of changes to which more than 20 women responded and concomitant self-care actions were as follows: (a) physical changes: vaginal dryness—"use lubricants" and "decrease douching"; (b) cognitive changes: forgetfulness/memory loss— "write notes; make lists; keep a log" and "do word puzzles to keep my mind active"; (c) personal changes: increased sense of freedom—"I introduce myself to people I want to get to know" and "tell others including my husband what I am going to do rather than asking permission"; (d) emotional changes: feelings of depression—"take hormones" and "I sing or do something I enjoy"; (e) psychological changes: staying asleep/going back to sleep—"think pleasant thoughts" and "drink a cup of herbal tea"; (f) vasomotor changes: hot flashes—"take tranquilizers" and "imagine the heat going out through my hands"; and (g) relationship changes: changes in roles with parents/significant others —"read about aging" and "give myself permission not to visit (parents) as much."

Health Deviation: Women identified 664 self-care actions related to health-deviation requisites, with an average of 4.3 ($SD = 2.3$). Frequencies and percentages of these actions are presented in Table 2. A majority of actions were related to routine care and diagnostic

Table 3. Stepwise Multiple Regression Analyses of Demographic Factors Contributing Significantly to Variance in Classified Self-Care Actions

Dependent Variable Predictor Variable	Beta	R	R^2	F
Universal Education	.29**	.29	.08	12.11**
Developmental Change				
Education	.28**	.25	.06	9.06*
Age	.25*	.35	.12	9.69**
Health Deviation				
Number of Children	-.28**	.24	.06	8.49*
Age	.24*	.34	.11	8.76**

$* p < .01;$ $** p < .001$

tests. Mammography was viewed by the majority of women as a way to promote well-being. Selected homeopathic remedies and meditation were self-care actions used for symptom care. Although the women in the study were self-defined and investigator-validated as healthy, the average number of chronic illnesses was .73 ($SD = .91$), with arthritis and hypertension most frequently identified. Many responses suggested actions performed for health as structural-functional integrity; however, when questioned, the women reaffirmed that the actions were performed to promote well-being, as defined for the study. Only 36 responses could not be classified as actions related to universal, developmental, or health-deviation self-care requisites.

Correlations among the nine categories of universal requisites, developmental change requisites, and health-deviation requisites showed universal elimination had the strongest relationship with developmental change, $r = .38$ ($p < .001$). Other significant moderate relationships ($p < .001$) between the developmental change category and the universal requisites were social interaction ($r = .35$), solitude ($r = .33$), and normalcy (self-esteem and self-image) ($r = .31$).

Low to low-moderate significant correlations were found between education and frequency of actions related to six universal self-care requisites, ranging from a low ($r = .19$) for hazards to a high ($r = .30$) for social interaction and normalcy. Three stepwise multiple regression analyses were also conducted. The number of actions performed in relationship to each of three types of requisites, universal, developmental change, and health deviation, were dependent variables for the analyses. Age, perception of middle age, race, religion, marital status, employment, number of children, dependency index (number of persons for whom the woman was financially, emotionally, or physically responsible), hours per week of employment, and income were predictor variables. Religion, marital status, and employment were dummycoded. Table 3 presents the summary of the regression analyses. Education explained 8% and 6% of the variance in frequency of actions related to the universal and developmental self-care requisites, respectively. Age contributed an additional 6% in explaining the variance in frequency of actions related to the developmental requisites. For the actions related to health deviation self-care requisites, number of children explained 6% of the variance and age contributed an additional 5% to the explained variance. All standardized regression coefficients were significant beyond the .01 level, with all variables contributing about equally to the prediction of frequency of self-care action.

Discussion

Healthy middle-aged women were knowledgeable about self-care actions that promote well-being and could readily articulate the information to interviewers. Women effortlessly described the actions and persuasively distinguished them from those performed to promote health as structural-functional integrity. Although the ability of women to identify self-care performed to promote well-being was anticipated from the pilot study and from the literature (Kolanowski & Gunter, 1985), the magnitude of responses was unanticipated. No other study on self-care or on health behaviors has generated the number and diversity of self-care actions.

The universal category of activity had the highest frequency of all self-care actions and included the four subcategories of physical exercise, talents/interests, religious and spiritual, and intellectual. Although not particular to middle-aged women, the religious and spiritual nature of self-care actions was supported by other self-care studies (Kolanowski & Gunter, 1985). The findings suggest that many women have some type of spiritual outreach, through organized religious activities or through experiencing nature. Many women identified physical actions performed for well-being, such as walking. However, the purpose was not only to meet the need for physical activity, but also to meet the need for solitude/social interaction and for outdoor air. Although others have identified the frequency of engagement in physical exercise by adults (Harris & Guten, 1979; Laffrey, 1983), few studies have explored multiple reasons for a single action.

Self-care actions related to social interaction were the second most frequently identified category within the universal type. Women took deliberate action to engage in social connectedness through contacts with friends and family members and performing many "helping" behaviors. Their engagement in actions related to interpersonal support has been suggested by other studies (Freer, 1980; Moore & Gaffney, 1989; Walker, Volkan, Sechrist, & Pender, 1988). When Kolanowski and Gunter (1985) explored the health patterns that promote well-being in retired career women, the most frequently identified actions were communicating and interacting with family members and social groups. The results from this study support these previous findings.

In contrast to many other studies of health behaviors in which nutrition and dietary actions were of primary importance to physical health (Flaskerud & Rush, 1989; Harris & Guten, 1979; Hautmann & Harrison, 1982; Laffrey, 1990), the women in this study identified actions related to nutrition/diet as the third most frequently performed self-care actions for well-being. The findings from a study of adults using a closed-ended questionnaire developed by Walker et al. (1988) suggested that these actions were important to health promotion. In contrast, Kolanowski and Gunter (1985) found that older women did not identify actions related to intake of food and beverages as promoting well-being. It could be that actions to meet the universal requisite for food are more important to promoting health, as structural and functional integrity, than to promoting well-being. However, actions associated with the pleasurable intake of food may be more relevant to promoting well-being.

When universal categories were divided into subcategories, the one with the highest frequency was prevention of hazards. Women were creative in their actions to feel safe in their environments, from methods of relating to people (to prevent violence) to physical safety, such as wearing seatbelts. Preventing hazards through creative, diverse methods to promote well-being was an unexpected finding. However, the frequency of actions in this category may have been related to a methodological flaw in the hazards questions, in which wearing seatbelts and locking doors were used as examples.

The importance of self-care actions to meet developmentally specific needs was evident from the number of actions performed to meet developmental self-care requisites. Almost 2000 of these were performed in response to specific changes that the women had experienced since turning 40. Many positive actions, such as those performed to enhance the change of "self-reflection," were identified, suggesting women's knowledge of self and ways to enhance well-being are deliberately performed as self-care. Although analysis of the relationship between specific developmental changes, such as hot flashes, and universal self-care requisites was not proposed for the study, significant findings suggest further investigation. With the strongest relationship between the self-care actions related to the universal self-care requisite of elimination and the developmental change requisite, the specific needs for personal hygiene and elimination during middle age become evident. Multiple individual examples of self-care actions associated with personal hygiene were listed, such as wearing panty liners and special bathing due to increased odors with middle age. These actions had been initiated since turning forty and were performed to promote well-being. The magnitude of the relationship between social interaction and the developmental change requisites supported the complexity of women's lives, with deliberate actions to maintain contact with parents, children, and friends. The relationship between self-care actions performed for the universal requisite of solitude and developmental changes suggested that women who perform many actions to promote solitude also act to meet developmental changes.

An unexpected finding was the importance of diagnostic testing to well-being. Although annual examinations and diagnostic testing, such as mammograms, are generally considered illness prevention, many of the women in this study performed the actions to improve their well-being. When interviewers questioned if the action was performed for their physical health or for well-being, the women verified the importance of the action to their well-being.

The interrelationship of the self-care requisites, or purposes for which self-care is performed, was an additional finding. As classification of action was not by the nature of the action alone, but by purpose for which it was performed, one action such as reading could be classified as meeting several needs or requisites; for example, activity (talents/interest or intellectual stimulation), rest (for relaxation), solitude (for escape), and normalcy (for self-concept). The multidimensional nature of the purposes for which actions are performed was described by Laffrey and Isenberg (1983) as reflecting the reality of individuals as complex beings. In the current study, each self-care action and concomitant purpose became the unit of analysis. However, the decision rules were restrictive and may have created ambiguous findings. For example, an action such as singing in the church choir was performed to meet the requisites of talents/interests/spiritual within the activity requisite, as well as those of social interaction and promotion of self-concept through normalcy. To separate out one action as meeting several distinct purposes may have been artificial, as, in reality, the purposes may be interrelated.

The overall variance explained by demographic factors on types of self-care actions was small, with none accounting for more than 12% of the variance. Women with higher levels of formal education tended to perform more self-care actions related to the universal self-care requisites of activity, solitude, social interaction, hazards, and normalcy, with social interaction and normalcy having the greatest magnitude. Women with more education also performed more activities related to the developmental changes and to health-deviation self-care requisites. Calnan (1985) found a similar relationship between level of education and frequency of both preventive and promotive health practices of middle-aged English women.

Almost without exception, as women described their own performance of self-care actions to promote well-being, their interest and level of involvement in recalling their deliberate actions increased. This enthusiasm for well-being as a component of overall health by women was supported by Woods et al. (1988).

The findings suggest that women have knowledge of self and of numerous, creative, and diverse self-care actions that promote their individual well-being. Whether learned within the context of formal education, shared through the generations, or learned through self-reflection, their impressive knowledge of individual self-care and their ability for recall supports a new view of the role of nurses in determining the needs of individual healthy women, that is, prescription of what needs to be done to promote well-being in the individual. In contrast to the nurse as the knowledge expert, the nurse can assist the woman to develop and enhance those actions that comprise the woman's identified self-care system. However, the personal and complex nature of the individual's self-care system must be acknowledged.

Accepted for publication February 11, 1993.
This research was supported in part by a grant from Illinois Wesleyan University and the Theta Pi and Lambda Chapters of Sigma Theta Tau International. The author gratefully acknowledges the conceptual/methodological guidance of Mary J. Denyes, PhD, RD, Wayne State University, and the computer programming/statistical support of Lisa Brown, PhD, and Teddy Amoloza, PhD, Illinois Wesleyan University.

Donna L. Hartweg, PhD, RN, is an associate professor and director of the School of Nursing, Illinois Wesleyan University, Bloomington, IL.

References

Calnan, M. (1985). Patterns in preventative behavior: A study of women in middle age. *Social Science Medicine, 20,* 263-268.

Dan, A., & Bernhard, L. A. (1989). Menopause and other health issues for midlife women. In S. Hunter, & M. Sundel (Eds.), *Midlife myths: Issues, findings, and practice implications* (pp. 51-63). Newbury Park: Sage.

Davidson, J. U. (1988). *Health embodiment: The relationship between self-care agency and health-promoting behaviors.* Unpublished doctoral dissertation, Texas Women's University, Denton, TX.

Flaskerud, J., & Rush, C. (1989). AIDS and traditional health beliefs and practices of Black women. *Nursing Research, 38,* 210-215.

Foster, M. (1987). *A study of the relationships among perceived current health, health-promoting activities and life satisfaction in older black adults.* Unpublished doctoral dissertation, University of Texas at Austin.

Freer, C. B. (1980). Self-care: A health diary study. *Medical Care, 18,* 853-861.

Germaine, L. M. (1984). *Behavioral treatment of menopausal hot flashes: Evaluation by objective methods (Heat stress, relaxation, flash provocation).* Unpublished doctoral dissertation, Wayne State University, Detroit.

Harris, D. M., & Guten, S. (1979). Health protective behavior: An exploratory study. *Journal of Health and Social Behavior, 20,* 17-29.

Hautmann, M., & Harrison, J. (1982). Health beliefs and practices in a middle-income Anglo-American neighborhood. *Advances in Nursing Science, 4,* 49-64.

Holsti, O. (1969). *Content analysis in the social sciences and humanities.* Reading, PA: Addison-Wesley.

Kolanowski, A., & Gunter, L. (1985). What are the health practices of retired career women? *Journal of Gerontological Nursing, 11*(12), 22-30.

Kulbok, P., & Baldwin, J. (1992). From preventive health behavior to health promotion: Advancing a positive construct of health. *Advances in Nursing Science, 14,* 50-64.

Laffrey, S. C. (1983). Health behavior choice as related to self-actualization, body weight, and health conception. *Dissertation Abstracts International 43,* 3536B.

Laffrey, S. C. (1990). An exploration of adult health behaviors. *Western Journal of Nursing Research, 12,* 434-447.

Laffrey, S. C., & Crabtree, M. K. (1988). Health and health behaviors of persons with chronic cardiovascular disease. *International Journal of Nursing Studies, 25*(1), 41-52.

Laffrey, S. C., & Isenberg, M. (1983). The relationship of internal locus of control, value placed on health, perceived importance of exercise, and participation in physical activity during leisure. *International Journal of Nursing Studies, 20*(3), 187-196.

Leiblum, S., Bachmann, G., Kemmann, E., Colburn, D., & Swartzman, L. (1983). Vaginal atrophy in the postmenopausal woman. *Journal of the American Medical Association, 249,* 2195-2198.

McElmurry, B., & Huddleston, D. (1991). Self-care and menopause: A critical review of research. *Health Care for Women International, 12*(1), 15-26.

Miles, M. B., & Huberman, A. M. (1984). Qualitative data analysis: A sourcebook for new methods. Beverly Hills, CA: Sage.

Moore, J. B., & Gaffney, K. F. (1989). Development of an instrument to measure mothers' performance of self-care activities for children. *Advances in Nursing Science, 12*(1), 76-84.

Neugarten, B. L. (1968). An awareness of middle age. In B. L. Neugarten (Ed.), *Middle age and aging: A reader on social psychology* (pp. 93-98). Chicago: University of Chicago.

Orem, D. E. (1991). *Nursing: Concepts of practice* (4th ed.). St. Louis: Mosby Year Book.

Pender, N. J. (1987). *Health promotion for nursing practice* (2nd ed.). Norwalk, CT: Appleton & Lang.

Prohaska, T., Leventhal, E., Leventhal, H., & Keller, M. (1985). Health practices and illness cognition in young, middle-aged, and elderly adults. *Journal of Gerontology, 40,* 569-578.

Riffle, K. L., Yoho, J., & Sams, J. (1989). Health-promoting behaviors, perceived social support, and self-reported health of Appalachian elderly. *Public Health Nursing, 6,* 204-211.

Stevenson, D. W., & Delprato, D. J. (1983). Multiple component of self-control program for menopausal hot flashes. *Journal of Behavioral Psychology, 14,* 137-140.

Voda, A. M. (1981). Climacteric hot flash. *Maturitas, 3,* 73-90.

Walker, S. N., Sechrist, K. R., & Pender, N. J. (1987). The health promoting life style profile: Development and psychometric characteristics. *Nursing Research, 36,* 76-81.

Walker, S. N., Volkan, K., Sechrist, K. R., & Pender, N. J. (1988). Health-promoting life styles of older adults: Comparisons with young and middle-aged adults, correlates and patterns. *Advances in Nursing Science, 11*(1), 76-90.

Woods, N. F. (1985). Self-care practices among young adult married women. *Research in Nursing and Health, 8,* 227-233.

Woods, N. F., Laffrey, S., Duffy, M., Lentz, M. J., Mitchell, E. S., Taylor, D., & Cowan, K. A. (1988). Being healthy: Women's images. *Advances in Nursing Science, 11*(2), 36-46.